Current Update on Foot and Ankle Arthroscopy

Editor

SEAN T. GRAMBART

CLINICS IN PODIATRIC MEDICINE AND SURGERY

www.podiatric.theclinics.com

Consulting Editor
THOMAS ZGONIS

October 2016 • Volume 33 • Number 4

ELSEVIER

1600 John F. Kennedy Boulevard • Suite 1800 • Philadelphia, Pennsylvania, 19103-2899

http://www.theclinics.com

CLINICS IN PODIATRIC MEDICINE AND SURGERY Volume 33, Number 4
October 2016 ISSN 0891-8422, ISBN-13: 978-0-323-46333-1

Editor: Jennifer Flynn-Briggs
Developmental Editor: Alison Swety

Clinics in Podiatric Medicine and Surgery (ISSN 0891-8422) is published quarterly by Elsevier Inc., 360 Park Avenue South, New York, NY 10010-1710. Months of issue are January, April, July, and October. Business and Editorial Offices: 1600 John F. Kennedy Blvd., Ste. 1800, Philadelphia, PA 19103-2899. Customer Service Office: 3251 Riverport Lane, Maryland Heights, MO 63043. Periodicals postage paid at New York, NY and additional mailing offices. Subscription prices are $285.00 per year for US individuals, $498.00 per year for US institutions, $100.00 per year for US students and residents, $370.00 per year for Canadian individuals, $602.00 for Canadian institutions, $435.00 for international individuals, $602.00 per year for international institutions and $220.00 per year for Canadian and foreign students/residents. To receive student/resident rate, orders must be accompanied by name of affiliated institution, date of term, and the *signature* of program/residency coordinator on institution letterhead. Orders will be billed at individual rate until proof of status is received. Foreign air speed delivery is included in all *Clinics* subscription prices. All prices are subject to change without notice. POSTMASTER: Send address changes to *Clinics in Podiatric Medicine and Surgery*, Elsevier Health Sciences Division, Subscription Customer Service, 3251 Riverport Lane, Maryland Heights, MO 63043. **Customer Service: 1-800-654-2452 (US). From outside of the US, call 314-447-8871. Fax: 314-447-8029. E-mail: JournalsCustomerService-usa@elsevier.com (for print support); JournalsOnlineSupport-usa@elsevier.com (for online support).**

Reprints. For copies of 100 or more of articles in this publication, please contact the Commercial Reprints Department, Elsevier Inc., 360 Park Avenue South, New York, NY 10010-1710. Tel.: 212-633-3874; Fax: 212-633-3820; E-mail: reprints@elsevier.com.

Clinics in Podiatric Medicine and Surgery is covered in *MEDLINE/PubMed (Index Medicus)* and *EMBASE/Excerpta Medica*.

CLINICS IN PODIATRIC MEDICINE AND SURGERY

CONSULTING EDITOR
THOMAS ZGONIS, DPM, FACFAS

Contributors

CONSULTING EDITOR

THOMAS ZGONIS, DPM, FACFAS
Professor and Director, Externship and Reconstructive Foot and Ankle Surgery Fellowship Programs, Division of Podiatric Medicine and Surgery, Department of Orthopaedics, University of Texas Health Science Center San Antonio, San Antonio, Texas

EDITOR

SEAN T. GRAMBART, DPM, FACFAS
President, American College of Foot and Ankle Surgeons, Department of Orthopedics, Carle Physician Group, Champaign, Illinois

AUTHORS

KEITH ARBUCKLE, DPM, AACFAS
Weil Foot & Ankle Institute, Chicago, Illinois

JOHN BACA, DPM, AACFAS
Weil Foot & Ankle Institute, Chicago, Illinois

JOSEPH S. BAKER, DPM, AACFAS
Fellow, Florida Orthopedic Foot and Ankle Center, Sarasota, Florida

ERIC A. BARP, DPM, FACFAS
The Iowa Clinic, West Des Moines, Iowa

LAURA BOHMAN, DPM
Department of Surgery, Cambridge Health Alliance, Harvard Medical School, Cambridge, Massachusetts

ZAC CAVINS, DPM
Podiatric Medicine and Surgery Resident (PGY1), Residency Training Program, Florida Hospital East Orlando, Orlando, Florida

JAMES M. COTTOM, DPM, FACFAS
Fellowship Director and Attending Surgeon, Florida Orthopedic Foot and Ankle Center, Sarasota, Florida

JOHN G. ERICKSON, DPM
UnityPoint Health, Des Moines, Iowa

ZACHARY FARLEY, DPM
Reconstructive Foot and Ankle Surgery, Orlando Foot and Ankle Clinic, Orlando, Florida

SEAN T. GRAMBART, DPM, FACFAS
President, American College of Foot and Ankle Surgeons, Department of Orthopedics, Carle Physician Group, Champaign, Illinois

BYRON HUTCHINSON, DPM, FACFAS
Medical Director, Franciscan Foot & Ankle Institute; Medical Director, Foot & Ankle Services Franciscan Health System; Franciscan Foot & Ankle Associates, Highline Clinic, Seattle, Washington

TREVOR PAYNE, DPM
Podiatric Medicine and Surgery Resident (PGY3), Residency Training Program, Florida Hospital East Orlando, Orlando, Florida

RONALD G. RAY, DPM, FACFAS, WCC, PT
Foot and Ankle Clinic of Montana, Affiliate, Great Falls Clinic, Great Falls, Montana

ERIC R. REESE, MS IV
Des Moines University, Des Moines, Iowa

CHRISTOPHER L. REEVES, DPM, FACFAS
Director of Research, Florida Hospital East Orlando Residency Training Program; Reconstructive Foot and Ankle Surgery, Orlando Foot and Ankle Clinic; Attending Physician, Surgical Residency Program, Department of Podiatric Surgery, Florida Hospital East Orlando, Orlando, Florida

AMBER M. SHANE, DPM, FACFAS
Reconstructive Foot and Ankle Surgery, Orlando Foot and Ankle Clinic; Attending Physician, Surgical Residency Program, Department of Podiatric Surgery, Florida Hospital East Orlando, Orlando, Florida

MATTHEW D. SORENSEN, DPM, FACFAS
Weil Foot & Ankle Institute, Chicago, Illinois

MICHAEL H. THEODOULOU, DPM, FACFAS
Instructor, Department of Surgery, Cambridge Health Alliance, Harvard Medical School, Cambridge, Massachusetts

RYAN VAZALES, DPM
Reconstructive Foot and Ankle Surgery, Orlando Foot and Ankle Clinic, Orlando, Florida

Contents

There are a number of variations in the intra-articular anatomy of the ankle which should not be considered pathological under all circumstances. The anteromedial corner of the tibial plafond (between the anterior edge of the tibial plafond and the medial malleolus) can have a notch, void of cartilage and bone. This area can appear degenerative arthroscopically; it is actually a normal variant of the articular surface. The anterior inferior tibiofibular ligament (AITF) can possess a lower, accessory band which can impinge on the anterolateral edge of the talar dome. In some cases it can cause irritation along this area of the talus laterally. If it is creating local irritation it can be removed since it does not provide any additional stabilization to the syndesmosis. There is a beveled region at the anterior leading edge of the lateral and dorsal surfaces of the talus laterally. This triangular region is void of cartilage and subchondral bone. The lack of talar structure in this region allows the lower portion of the AITF ligament to move over the talus during end range dorsiflexion of the ankle, preventing impingement. The variation in talar anatomy for this area should not be considered pathological.

In recent years, arthroscopic procedures of the foot and ankle have seen a significant increase in both indications and popularity. Furthermore, technological advances in video quality, fluid management, and other arthroscopy-specific instruments continue to make arthroscopic procedures more effective with reproducible outcomes. As surgeons continue to use this approach, it is important that they have a complete understanding of the instrumentation available to them, including their indications and limitations.

Arthroscopy of the ankle is used in the treatment and diagnosis of a spectrum of intra-articular pathology including soft tissue and osseous impingement, osteochondral lesions, arthrofibrosis, and synovitis. To help identify the correct pathology, imaging techniques are often used to aid the surgeon

foot function. Endoscopic debridement of the plantar fascia can be performed reproducibly to reduce pain and maintain function of the foot.

Arthroscopic lateral ankle stabilization procedures have been described for many years. New technological advances and a deeper understanding of the pathobiomechanics involved in chronic lateral ankle instability have allowed an expansion of arthroscopic approaches to this common pathology. As experience is gained and outcomes within the patient profile are understood, the authors feel that the arthroscopic approach to lateral ankle stabilization may prove superior to traditional methods secondary to the risk and traditional complications that are mitigated within minimally invasive arthroscopic approaches. Additionally, the arthroscopic approach may allow a quicker return to ballistic sport and decrease time for rehabilitation.

Arthroscopy has advanced in the foot and ankle realm, leading to new innovative techniques designed toward treatment of small joint abnormality. A range of abnormalities that are currently widespread for arthroscopic treatment in larger joints continues to be translated to congruent modalities in the small joints. Small joint arthroscopy offers relief from foot ailments with a noninvasive element afforded by arthroscopy. Early studies have found comparable results from arthroscopic soft tissue procedures as well as arthrodesis of the small joints when compared with the standard open approach.

Arthroscopic ankle arthrodesis is a cost-effective option for many patients with posttraumatic arthritis of the ankle joint. Rehabilitation is generally quicker than conventional open techniques, and rates of fusion are comparable or better than traditional open techniques. Unless the arthroscopic surgeon has considerable experience, the best results are seen in patients with very little deformity in the ankle joint.

CLINICS IN PODIATRIC MEDICINE AND SURGERY

FORTHCOMING ISSUES

January 2017
The Diabetic Charcot Foot and Ankle: A Multidisciplinary Team Approach
Thomas Zgonis, *Editor*

April 2017
Achilles Tendon Pathology
Paul D. Dayton, *Editor*

July 2017
Foot and Ankle Arthrodesis
John J. Stapleton, *Editor*

October 2017
Surgical Advances in Ankle Arthritis
Alan Ng, *Editor*

RECENT ISSUES

July 2016
Dermatological Manifestations of the Lower Extremity
Tracey C. Vlahovic, *Editor*

April 2016
Nerve-Related Injuries and Treatments for the Lower Extremity
Stephen L. Barrett, *Editor*

January 2016
Tendon Reconstruction and Transfers of the Foot and Ankle
Christopher L. Reeves, *Editor*

October 2015
Secondary Procedures in Total Ankle Replacement
Thomas S. Roukis, *Editor*

RELATED INTEREST

Foot and Ankle Clinics, June 2016 (Vol. 21, Issue 2)
New Ideas and Techniques in Foot and Ankle Surgery: A Global Perspective
John G. Anderson and Donald R. Bohay, *Editors*
Available at: http://www.foot.theclinics.com/

THE CLINICS ARE AVAILABLE ONLINE!
Access your subscription at:
www.theclinics.com

Foreword

Current Update on Foot and Ankle Arthroscopy

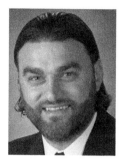

Thomas Zgonis, DPM, FACFAS
Consulting Editor

This issue of *Clinics in Podiatric Medicine and Surgery* is focused on the diagnosis and treatment of various foot and ankle conditions with arthroscopic surgery. Arthroscopic surgery of the foot and ankle can be used for a wide spectrum of soft tissue and osseous abnormality, including ankle ligamentous repair and ankle arthrodesis. This issue covers in detail the arthroscopic anatomy, medical imaging, and most common instrumentation utilized in arthroscopic surgery. A variety of topics from repair of posterior ankle impingement and lateral ankle stabilization to repair of talar osteochondral lesions and ankle arthrodesis are very well reviewed by our guest editor, Dr Grambart, and invited authors.

A thorough preoperative history, physical examination, and medical imaging along with proper understanding of anatomic landmarks and portals, surgical patient positioning, type of anesthesia, and knowledge of arthroscopic instrumentation are paramount for the patient's overall successful outcome. In conclusion, I would like to thank our guest editor, Dr Grambart, invited authors, editorial board, and all of our readers for their outstanding submissions and continuous support of *Clinics in Podiatric Medicine and Surgery*.

Thomas Zgonis, DPM, FACFAS
Division of Podiatric Medicine and Surgery
Department of Orthopaedics
University of Texas Health
Science Center San Antonio
7703 Floyd Curl Drive, MSC 7776
San Antonio, TX 78229, USA

E-mail address:
zgonis@uthscsa.edu

Clin Podiatr Med Surg 33 (2016) xi
http://dx.doi.org/10.1016/j.cpm.2016.08.002
0891-8422/16/© 2016 Published by Elsevier Inc.

podiatric.theclinics.com

Preface

Arthroscopy of the Foot and Ankle

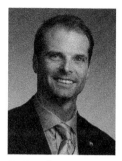

Sean T. Grambart, DPM, FACFAS
Editor

The evolution of foot and ankle arthroscopy continues to advance over the years. I have had the privilege of participating as faculty at the American College of Foot and Ankle Surgeons arthroscopy course over the last several years. It is amazing how quickly the surgeons attending the course advance with their arthroscopic skills. The residents that attend the course are exposed to much more arthroscopic technique than what I was exposed to as a resident. I remember taking that course when I was a resident, and I know I did not have the technique that the surgeons have now. This is a credit to the profession and the surgeons that continue to find ways to advance techniques and procedures and pass those teachings on to others.

As our arthroscopic skills advance, so does our need for better instrumentation and research on outcomes for arthroscopic procedures. This *Clinics in Podiatric Medicine and Surgery* allows the authors to showcase some of the newer techniques and some of the "gold-standard" techniques that still stand the test of time. I believe that this issue of *Clinics in Podiatric Medicine and Surgery* is relevant to all skill sets. There are articles that will take the reader from arthroscopic anatomy and instrumentation all the way to ankle arthrodesis and endoscopic plantar fascia debridement, for example.

I would like to thank all of the authors that have contributed to this issue of *Clinics in Podiatric Medicine and Surgery*. It has been a privilege working with them and seeing their expertise in the world of arthroscopy. They have given up their time and have

Clin Podiatr Med Surg 33 (2016) xiii–xiv
http://dx.doi.org/10.1016/j.cpm.2016.08.001
0891-8422/16/© 2016 Published by Elsevier Inc.

contributed their knowledge and skills in the hopes that this issue of *Clinics in Podiatric Medicine and Surgery* is useful and enjoyable to the readers.

Sean T. Grambart, DPM, FACFAS
Carle Physician Group
1802 South Mattis Avenue
Champaign, IL, 61821, USA

E-mail address:
sean.grambart@carle.com

Arthroscopic Anatomy of the Ankle Joint

Ronald G. Ray, DPM, WCC, PT

KEYWORDS

- Ankle anatomy • Intra-articular ankle anatomy • Anatomy of tibial plafond
- Anatomy lateral mallelous • Talar anatomy

KEY POINTS

- The anteromedial corner of the tibial plafond has a notch of variable size that is void of cartilage and is considered a normal variant of the articular surface.
- The anterior inferior tibiofibular ligament can have a low-lying band that can normally impinge on the anterolateral border of the talus.
- The deep transverse ligament of the posterior inferior tibiofibular ligament is considered a true labrum of the ankle joint and has been implicated in posterior ankle impingement.
- The anterior talofibular ligament and components of the deltoid ligament are intracapsular, but extrasynovial and not easily visualized arthroscopically.

Arthroscopy of the ankle joint provides a highly accurate means of locating and treating intra-articular abnormality. It is imperative to have a sound appreciation of the intra-articular environment of the normal ankle joint. This discussion focuses on the anatomic structures of the ankle joint that can be visualized through the arthroscope.

OSSEOUS STRUCTURES OF THE ANKLE JOINT

The ankle joint is composed of the tibia and fibula superiorly and the talus inferiorly. The distal aspect of the tibia is composed (from medial to lateral) of the medial malleolus, the tibial plafond, and the nonarticular lateral surface. The medial malleolus has an anterior, inferior, medial, posterior, and lateral surface. It is possible to visualize a large portion of the medial malleolus arthroscopically. The anterior aspect of the medial malleolus has a flat to slightly domed surface from medial to lateral. The anterior surface is flat to slightly convex from superior to inferior. The inferior aspect of the medial malleolus has 2 protruberances or colliculi, anterior and posterior. The former extends more inferiorly (by 0.5 cm) than the latter, with an intervening intercollicular groove.[1] The deep anterior and posterior tibiotalar ligaments of the deltoid arise from the

Foot and Ankle Clinic of Montana, Affiliate, Great Falls Clinic, 1301 11th Avenue South, Suite 6, Great Falls, MT 59405, USA
E-mail address: drronray@q.com

Clin Podiatr Med Surg 33 (2016) 467–480
http://dx.doi.org/10.1016/j.cpm.2016.06.001
0891-8422/16/$ – see front matter © 2016 Elsevier Inc. All rights reserved.

podiatric.theclinics.com

anterior and posterior colliculi, respectively.[1] It is possible to visualize the medial surface of the medial malleolus above the inferior margins of the colliculi. The posterior surface of the medial malleolus cannot be visualized arthroscopically from within the ankle joint. In its upper one-half, this surface is slightly convex, whereas in the lower one-half, this surface becomes concave or grooved to accommodate the passage of the posterior tibial tendon. The lateral surface of the medial malleolus is comma-shaped and covered with cartilage to articulate with the medial articular facet of the talus (**Fig. 1**).[1] The cartilage on this surface can be seen to extend onto the margin or border of the anterior and inferior surfaces of the medial malleolus (**Fig. 2**).

The inferior surface of the tibia or tibial plafond is covered with hyaline cartilage to articulate with the talar dome. The surface is concave from anterior to posterior. The anterior and lateral borders are wider than the posterior and medial borders. Looking from below, the surface is somewhat rhomboid shaped with the base lateral and the upper narrower surface facing medially (**Fig. 3**). The posterior margin of the tibial plafond extends more inferiorly than the anterior margin. The more inferior position of the posterior tibial margin places the posterior capsular structures in a more inferior position, making them more difficult to visualize through standard anterolateral and anteromedial portals. Visualization of structures in the posterior aspect of the ankle joint is further complicated by the amount of coverage the tibial plafond provides over the talar articular surface. Regardless of the position of the talus (dorsiflexion or plantarflexion), two-thirds of the talar surface is always covered by the tibial plafond, leaving only one-third uncovered at all times.[1,2]

A variation in the osseous and/or cartilaginous surface of the anterior medial tibial plafond requires further comment. The junction between the anterior medial margin of the tibia and the superior lateral margin of the medial malleolus marks the location of a posteriorly directed void or notch. The apparent defect represents either an isolated loss of cartilage or an absence of both cartilage and underlying bone (**Figs. 4** and **5**). Ray and colleagues[3] found this area of deficit to represent a normal variation in the articular surface of the anterior medial tibial plafond. This region was not associated with degenerative changes in 77 specimens. The investigators noted that in 12 of 62 (19%) specimens, the capsule or synovial lining of the ankle joint attached to and followed the articular margins of the notch. In 32 others (52%), a capsular

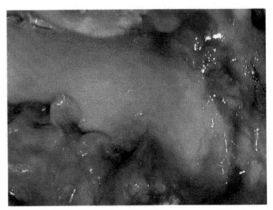

Fig. 1. Lateral aspect medial malleolus, right ankle. A view looking from lateral to medial at the comma-shaped lateral articular surface of the medial malleolus. Notice the anterior colliculus extends more inferiorly than the posterior colliculus.

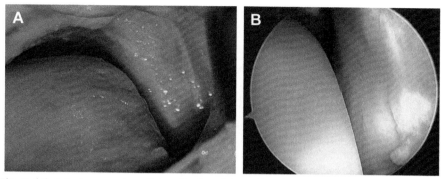

Fig. 2. (*A*) Anterior aspect medial malleolus, right ankle. The talus is on the left; the medial malleolus is on the right. Notice the articular surface extends onto the anterior aspect of the malleolus. (*B*) Arthroscopic image of the medial malleolus and medial gutter, right ankle. The talus is on the left, and the medial malleolus on the right. The medial joint line is aligned vertically. Cartilage can be seen extending onto the anterior aspect of the medial malleolus.

reflection was found to follow the shape of the notch but not have attachment to it. In the final 18 specimens (29%), the capsule did not follow the outline of the notch.[3] A recent MRI investigation evaluated the anteromedial aspect of the tibia in 106 patients who underwent MRI of the ankle. The notch was identified in 48 of 106 patients or 45% (24 males and 24 female patients). The average size of the notch was 6.2 mm ± 1.5 mm in width and 1.2 mm ± 0.5 mm in depth. The notch was considered prominent in only 6 patients. None of the patients with a notch demonstrated any signal changes consistent with either the presence of edema or cystic change.[4]

The lateral surface of the tibia is a triangular-shaped depression with its apex facing superiorly and the base inferior. The inferior margin of the triangle is covered in cartilage allowing it to articulate with a similarly shaped articular surface on the medial aspect of the fibula.[5,6] The union of the tibia and the fibula at this location creates the syndesmotic recess (**Fig. 6**). In some cases, a small fringe of soft tissue can be seen extruding out from the recess.

Three surfaces of the lateral malleolus can be visualized arthroscopically: lateral, anterior, and medial. The lateral surface is convex and can only be seen arthroscopically anteriorly, where it meets the anterior surface of the fibula. The anterior surface of the fibular malleolus slopes posteriorly, from superior to its broad apex inferiorly (**Fig. 7**).

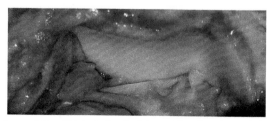

Fig. 3. Inferior surface of the tibial plafond, right ankle. The tibial plafond is wider anteriorly and laterally. It is narrower medially and posteriorly. Also notice the central portion of the anterior margin of the tibia extends more inferiorly than the rest of the anterior edge.

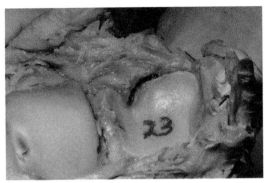

Fig. 4. The anteromedial tibial notch or pseudonotch of Hardy. View of the tibial plafond from below of a left ankle. The talus is rotated to the left of the image; the fibula is to the right. Notice the capsular reflection following the contour of the margins of the tibial notch.

The lower medial surface of the fibular malleolus has a triangular facet with its base facing superiorly and its apex extending inferiorly.[1] The surface is convex from anterior to posterior and even more so from superior to inferior; this allows it to match the lateral triangular surface of the talus (**Fig. 8**). The fibula can be seen to extend more distally in a vertical orientation beyond the triangular convex articular surface.

Surfaces of the talus that are visible during ankle arthroscopy include the dorsal, medial, lateral, and talar neck (medially, dorsally, and laterally). The dorsal articular surface, or talar dome, is convex from anterior to posterior, wider anteriorly, and narrower posteriorly. The variation in the transverse distance between the anterior and posterior surfaces of the talus is as low as 2.4 mm $\pm$ 1.3 mm.[2] In a separate investigation, the mean transverse width difference was 4.2 mm with a minimum variation in width of 2 mm and a maximum variation in width of 6 mm.[1,7,8] In 80% of tali, there is a sagittal (longitudinal) groove or depression running from anterior to posterior, biased slightly more toward the medial aspect of the dorsal surface (**Fig. 9**). In the remaining 20% of tali, the longitudinal depression takes on a more complex shape

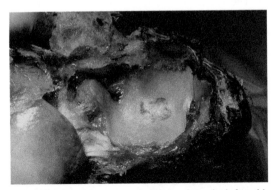

Fig. 5. The anteromedial tibial notch or pseudonotch of Hardy, left ankle. View of the tibial plafond from below in a left ankle. In this specimen, the notch has no capsular or synovial reflections following its outline. Also notice how the articular margins are sharp, without fibrillation or degenerative changes.

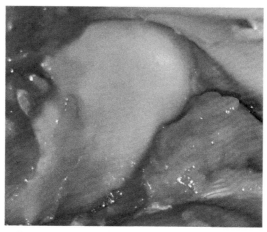

Fig. 6. The syndesmotic recess, right ankle. View of the syndesmosis with the talus removed. Notice how tightly the fibula fits against the tibia.

with a concavity on the medial aspect and more of a convexity on the lateral aspect. The tibial plafond will have a surface that mirrors the unique shape of the dorsal talar surface.[1] The anterior articular margin of the talar surface can be variable in shape from straight, to convex, to concave. In the author's experience, the medial surface tends to extend more anteriorly onto the talar neck than the lateral surface, creating a reciprocal convex to concave margin from medial to lateral.

The articular cartilage of the talar dome can extend onto the talar neck either anteromedially or anterolaterally. These medial or lateral extensions of the articular surface should not be considered pathologic. The medial extension of the articular surface onto the anteromedial talar neck can be seen from 11% to 55% of ankles.[2,9–11] There

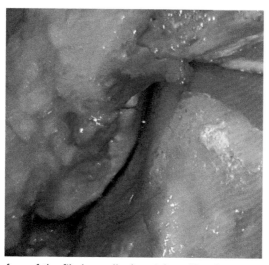

Fig. 7. Anterior surface of the fibular malleolus, right ankle. The articular surface medially will extend slightly onto the anterior surface. The lateral joint line is vertical superiorly and then angulates laterally in the lower one-half.

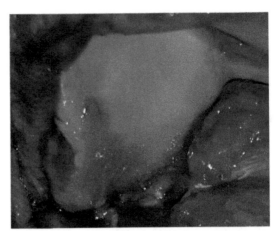

Fig. 8. The triangular, medial articular surface of the fibula, right ankle. Anterior is to the left; posterior is to the right. The proximal attachment of the calcaneofibular ligament arises from the inferior-posterior surface of the fibula, while the ATFL comes off the anterior-inferior surface.

will be an extension of the lateral articular surface of the medial malleolus to accompany the anterior extension of the talar articular surface onto the talar neck. A lateral extension of the articular surface onto the anterolateral aspect of the talar neck can be seen from 17% to 54.6% of ankles.[2,9,11]

The medial surface of the talus consists of an upper articular surface and a lower nonarticular portion. The upper articular component is in coverage by the reciprocal lateral surface of the medial malleolus (comma-shaped). The surface poses a wider (from dorsal to plantar), circular, articular facet anteriorly that is continuous with a narrower posterior portion.[1] The entire surface is comma-shaped, similar to the lateral surface of the medial malleolus. The posterior extent of the medial articular surface of the talus ends at the margin between medial and dorsal articular surfaces. The dorsal articular surface of the talar dome continues in a posterior direction beyond the termination of the medial articular surface (**Fig. 10**). The junction or shoulder area

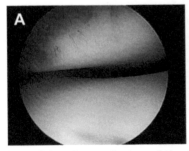
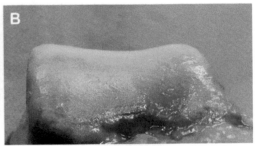

Fig. 9. (A) Arthroscopic view of the dorsal articular surface of the talus in a right ankle. Notice the dorsal surface is not flat but has a distinct central to a slightly medial sagittal groove or depression from anterior to posterior. (B) Anterior view of the talar dome, right ankle. The dorsal surface of the talus has a distinct sagittal groove located centrally or may be biased toward the medial aspect of the talus.

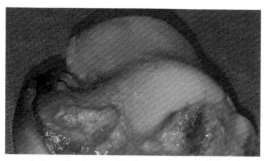

Fig. 10. Medial aspect of the talus in a right foot. The comma-shaped medial articular surface can be seen, wider from dorsal to plantar anteriorly and becoming narrower posteriorly. Note the dorsal articular surface continues beyond the posterior extent of the medial articular surface.

between the dorsal and medial articular surfaces of the talus is rounded or one-quarter dome-shaped (**Fig. 11**).

Not unlike the extension of the dorsal articular surface onto the dorsomedial aspect of the talar neck, the medial articular surface can extend onto the medial aspect of the talar neck as an articular extension. Extension of the medial surface onto the medial talar neck has been demonstrated 91% of the time, either in isolation or in conjunction with an anterior extension of the dorsal articular surface.[1]

The lateral surface of the talus is a triangular articular facet that possesses a convex dorsal margin that is in continuity with the dorsal articular surface of the talus. The surface extends vertically downward from its dorsal articular margin, becoming increasingly more concave inferiorly. The mean arc of curvature inferiorly measures 106 ± 13° (**Fig. 12**).[2,12] The junction or shoulder area between the dorsal and lateral articular surfaces has a sharper or 90° degree edge compared with the gentler, rounded, or dome-shaped medial talar shoulder.

There is a beveled area, void of cartilage, at the anterior-superior-most aspect of the lateral talar surface, where it meets the dorsal, anterior, lateral extent of the talar dome. Frequently, this beveled region is also void of subchondral or cortical bone. The angle of this bevel corresponds with the alignment of the lower-most band of the anterior inferior tibiofibular ligament (AITF) as it courses from the fibula to the tibia. During

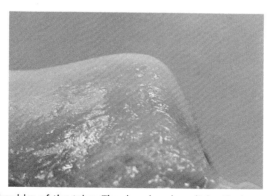

Fig. 11. Medial shoulder of the talus. The dorsal and medial articular surfaces of the talus meet at the medial shoulder. This area is rounded or has the shape of a one-quarter circle.

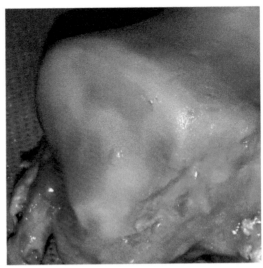

Fig. 12. Lateral surface of the talus in a right ankle. The surface is concave from superior to inferior and convex from anterior to posterior.

maximum ankle dorsiflexion, the lower-most band of the AITF (if it rides low enough) will travel directly in front of this beveled region on the talus. The lack of talar structure and volume in this area allows the ligament to travel uninterrupted during end-range dorsiflexion of the ankle (**Fig. 13**).[13]

A portion of the neck of the talus is found within the confines of the ankle joint capsule anteriorly. Overall, the talar neck extends anteromedially in a downward direction.[1] The dorsal aspect of the talar neck lies at a position inferior or lower than the

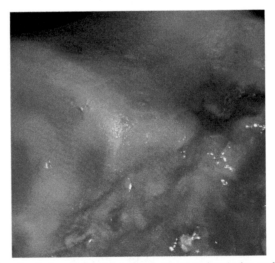

Fig. 13. Beveled region between the lateral and dorsal and articular surfaces of the talus. This region is void of cartilage and cortical bone, leaving the cancellous bone exposed. This region accommodates the passage of the AITF during end range dorsiflexion.

anterior extent of the dorsal articular surface of the talar dome. When the neck takes up a position below the surface of the talar dome, the tibia is less likely to impinge on the neck during end-range dorsiflexion of the ankle. Because of the external rotation of the talar head and neck in relation to the talar body, the dorsal surface of the talar neck tends to incline from lateral to medial. Because of this inclination of the neck from lateral to medial, the dropoff (or height) from the anterior extent of the talar dome to the dorsal aspect of the talar neck is greater laterally and gets progressively less in a medial direction.

CAPSULAR ATTACHMENTS OF THE ANKLE JOINT

The intra-articular volume of the ankle joint is defined by the joint capsule, which is lined by a single layer of synovium in the normal state. Beginning medially, the capsule attaches along the medial aspect of the talar body below the medial articular facet and above the tubercle of insertion of the deltoid ligament.[6] Posteriorly, the capsule is quite thin, blending with the fibers of the deep transverse ligament (DTL) of the posterior inferior tibiofibular ligament (PITF). Laterally, the capsule follows the contours of the triangular articular surface on the talus and also follows the margins of the similarly shaped medial surface of the fibula. The posterior talofibular and anterior talofibular ligaments (ATFLs) create substantial thickening and enlargements of the joint capsule, posterolaterally and anterolaterally, respectively, but are not intercapsular.[5] Anterolaterally, the joint capsule extends anteriorly from the tip of the fibula, not following the anterior extent of the triangular lateral talar surface. Instead, the capsule proceeds directly anterior to the lateral aspect of the neck of the talus beyond the anterior extent of the articular surface of the talar dome. Once it reaches this anterior landmark, the capsule extends superiorly up the lateral aspect of the talar neck. The capsule then proceeds across the entire width of the talar neck to the medial side, anterior to the medial articular surface of the talus. There is a very distinct pouch or opening directly anterior to the anterior extent of the dorsal articular surface of the talar dome to prevent tibial impingement on the anterior capsule (**Fig. 14**).

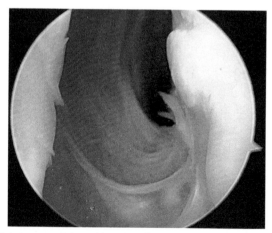

Fig. 14. Anterior joint space, right ankle. View from medial to lateral. The anterior leading edge of the talar dome is to the right. Notice the capsular space across the dorsal aspect of the talar neck.

Superiorly, the ankle joint capsule attaches to the distal tibial metaphysis at an average distance of 9.6 mm (4.9 mm to 27.0 mm) proximal to the anteroinferior tibial margin. Moving laterally, proximal to the tibiofibular recess, the average proximal extension of the capsule is 19.2 mm (12.7 mm to 38.0 mm).[14] Because the joint capsule attaches significantly proximal to the anterior joint line, it is possible to remove osseous spurs from the anterior margin of the tibia arthroscopically.

LIGAMENTOUS STRUCTURES FOUND WITHIN THE ANKLE JOINT

The ankle joint is stabilized by ligamentous structures found on all 4 sides of the ankle. Only 2 ligament complexes are truly intra-articular: the AITF and the PITF. The deltoid ligament, the ATFL, the calcaneofibular ligament, and the posterior talofibular ligament are considered "closely related" to the ankle joint capsule. In many cases, these ligaments are considered to be intra-capsular, but not intra-articular.[1,5,6]

The distal tibiofibular syndesmosis is stabilized by the AITF ligament, the interosseous ligament, and the PITF ligament (superficial and deep components). A syndesmotic recess is created inferiorly by the union of the tibia and fibula. The recess becomes a vertical extension of the tibiotalar joint space lined with synovium.[15] The recess is limited: (1) superiorly, by the inferior extent of the interosseous ligament; (2) posteriorly, by an attachment along the fibula posteriorly, superior to the triangular articular facet, as well as a broad attachment off the DTL (part of the PITF Ligament); and (3) anteriorly, by an attachment onto the anterior margin of the fibula superior to the medial articular facet of the fibula.[15] The entrance to the syndesmotic recess (from the tibiotalar joint) will commonly have a fold or redundancy of fatty synovial tissue easily visualized arthroscopically (**Fig. 15**). The redundant synovial tissue is made up of loose connective tissue intermixed with vessels and nerves.[16,17]

The AITF ligament is intra-articular within the ankle joint, providing stability to the anterior aspect of the distal or inferior tibiofibular syndesmosis. It arises from the anterior or leading edge of the tibia and extends inferiorly and laterally to insert onto the anterior border of the fibula.[1] The structure of the ligament consists of a varying number of bands that can take on a variety of configurations. In some cases, a lower band can be seen distinct from the upper portion of the ligament (**Fig. 16**).[13] Whether a distinct lower band exists or not, the lower margin of the ligament can be positioned

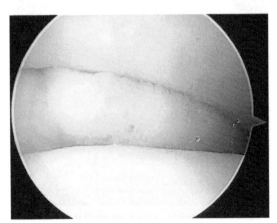

Fig. 15. Arthroscopic image of the synovial fold at the entrance to the syndesmotic recess found between the tibia and fibula.

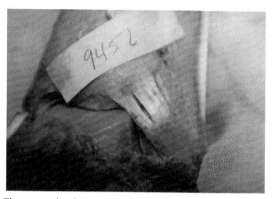

Fig. 16. The AITF. There can be 2 or more distinct bands to this ligament. Notice how an exceptionally low inferior band can rest or impinge on the talus. In some cases, the talus will have a beveled margin between the dorsal and lateral articular surfaces.

such that it will impinge on or rub against the lateral shoulder of the talus anteriorly. In some cases, where ligamentous impingement is present on the talus, the lateral shoulder of the talus anteriorly has a distinct beveled edge. This beveled edge should not be considered degenerative in nature, but rather, an anatomic variation of the articular surface to accommodate a low-lying AITF ligament.[13]

The PITF ligament provides stability to the posterior aspect of the syndesmosis. The PITF comprises 2 parts: superficial and deep. The superficial portion of the ligament is consistent in structure and function to its counterpart anteriorly, the AITF ligament. The superficial PITF arises from the posterolateral aspect of the posterior tubercle of the tibia. The fibers extend inferior, posterior, and lateral to insert on the posterior border of the fibula above the digital fossa of the lateral malleolus.[1,18,19] The inferior-most fibers of the superficial component of the ligament may be visible arthroscopically. The deep component of the PITF ligament has been given a variety of names, including inferior transverse ligament, DTL, transverse ligament, and inferior transverse portion of the PITF ligament.[1,6,18,19] The DTL arises from and inserts onto points just inferior to the attachments described for the superficial component of the PITF ligament (**Fig. 17**). The DTL articulates with the posterior articular surface of the talus and is

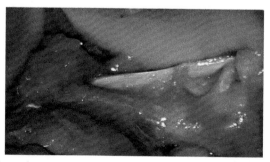

Fig. 17. Looking into the posterior aspect of a right ankle with the talus removed. The medial fibular articular surface is on the left. The lower fibers of the superficial PITF ligament are at the upper part of the image immediately between the fibula and tibia. The DLT is the white fibers coursing from lateral to medial in the center of the image.

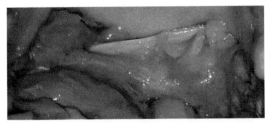

Fig. 18. Posterior aspect of a right ankle, talus removed. Below the DTL (white fibers coursing from left to right across image) is the IML coursing from lateral to medial.

considered a true labrum that deepens and stabilizes the posterior aspect of the joint.[18]

Coursing just below the DTL is the intermalleolar ligament (IML). The IML blends with the DTL at its tibial origin, but becomes separated from the DTL as it courses toward its extrasynovial fibular origin (**Fig. 18**).[18] During plantarflexion, the IML becomes less taut and approximates the DTL, making it more difficult to appreciate arthroscopically. Rosenberg and colleagues[20] identified the IML in 56% of the specimens they evaluated with 20% having 2 or 3 bands. In a separate cadaveric investigation, the IML was present in 72% of specimens with a mean length of 23.5 mm and a mean width of 4.0 mm.[21] The IML can be the cause of posterior ankle impingement.[22,23]

INTRACAPSULAR—EXTRASYNOVIAL LIGAMENTS OF THE ANKLE JOINT

The ATFL ligament arises from the anterior leading edge of the fibula and extends anteromedially to insert onto the talar body (at the base of the talar neck laterally), anterior to the lateral talar articular surface.[1,19] The ATFL will commonly have a wider upper band and a narrower lower band. Occasionally, another narrow, lower band can be observed.[1,21,24] The center of the fibular attachment of the ATFL is approximately 10 mm from the tip of the lateral malleolus. During ankle plantarflexion, the upper band

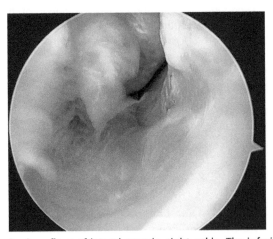

Fig. 19. Arthroscopic view, floor of lateral capsule, right ankle. The inferior talofibular surface is seen in the center of the image. The ATFL is found under the synovial lining extending from the anterior fibula toward the camera.

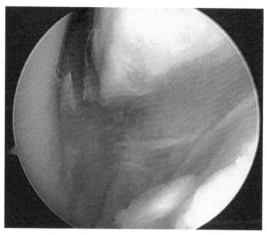

Fig. 20. Arthroscopic view, floor of medial capsule, right ankle. Capsular area below the medial malleolus. The capsule in this region is made up of the anterior tibiotalar fascicle.

of the ATFL becomes taut, whereas the lower band or bands become relaxed. Dorsiflexion of the ankle will cause the upper band to lose tension, whereas the lower band or bands become taut.[19] The ATFL is located outside the synovial lining of the joint. It can only be seen arthroscopically if the synovial lining is not exceptionally thickened or fibrosed (**Fig. 19**).

The deltoid ligament is primarily responsible for stabilizing the medial aspect of the ankle joint. Not unlike the ATFL, the deltoid ligament is considered intracapsular and extrasynovial. Portions of the deltoid ligament may be observed arthroscopically depending on the state of the synovial lining extending from the medial malleolus to the talar body and neck. The deltoid ligament has both superficial and deep components. The superficial deltoid includes anterior superficial tibiotalar fascicle, tibionavicular fascicle, tibiocalcaneal ligament, and superficial tibiotalar ligament. The deep deltoid includes deep anterior tibiotalar ligament, deep posterior tibiotalar ligament, and anterior tibiotalar fascicle.[1,25,26] The anterior tibiotalar fascicle will make up the floor of the ankle capsule, extending from the medial malleolus to the medial aspect of the talar neck/head (**Fig. 20**).[1] Inferior and posterior to the medial malleolus, portions of the deep anterior and posterior tibiotalar ligaments make-up the capsular structure and are synovial lined.

REFERENCES

1. Sarafian SK. Anatomy of the foot and ankle: descriptive topographic, functional. 2nd edition. Philadelphia: J. B. Lippincott Company; 1993. p. 37–112, 159–217.
2. Inman VT. The joints of the ankle. Baltimore (MD): Williams & Wilkins; 1976.
3. Ray RG, Gusman DN, Christensen JC. Anatomical variation of the tibial plafond: the anteromedial tibial notch. J Foot Ankle Surg 1994;33(4):419–26.
4. Boutin RD, Chang J, Bateni C, et al. The notch of harty (pseudodefect of the tibial plafond): frequency and characteristic findings at MRI of the ankle. AJR Am J Roentgenol 2015;205(2):358–63.
5. Gray H. Anatomy of the human body. 9th edition. Philadelphia: Lea & Febiger; 1973. p. 247–58, 355–60.

6. Draves D. Anatomy of the lower extremity. Baltimore (MD): Williams & Wilkins; 1986. p. 72–9, 107–12.
7. Testut L. 7th edition. Traite d'anatomie humaine, vol. 1. Paris: Doin; 1921. p. 632.
8. Poirier P, Charpy A. Traite d'anatomie humaine, vol. 1. Paris: Masson; 1899. p. 758.
9. Singh I. Squatting facets on the talus and tibia in Indians. J Anat 1959;93:540.
10. Sewell RBS. A study of the astragalus: III. The collum tali. J Anat Physiol 1906;39: 74.
11. Barnett CH. Squatting facets on the European talus. J Anat 1954;88:509.
12. Barnett CH, Napier JR. The axis of rotation at the ankle joint in man: its influence upon the form of the talus and its mobility of the fibula. J Anat 1952;86:1.
13. Ray RG, Kriz BM. Anterior inferior tibiofibular ligament: variations and relationship to the talus. J Am Podiatr Med Assoc 1991;81(9):479–85.
14. Lee PT, Clarke MT, Bearcroft PW, et al. The proximal extent of the ankle capsule and safety for insertion of percutaneous fine wires. J Bone Joint Surg Br 2005; 87(5):668–71.
15. Hermans JJ, Beumer A, de Jong TA, et al. Anatomy of the distal tibiofibular syndesmosis in adults: a pictorial essay with a multimodality approach. J Anat 2010; 217(6):633–45.
16. Bartonicek J. Anatomy of the tibiofibular syndesmosis and its clinical relevance. Surg Radiol Anat 2003;25:379–86.
17. Kim S, Huh YM, Song HT, et al. Chronic tibiofibular syndesmosis injury of ankle: evaluation with contrast-enhanced fat-suppressed 3D fast spoiled gradient-recalled acquisition in the steady state MR imaging. Radiology 2007;242:225–35.
18. Golanó P, Mariani PP, Rodríguez-Niedenfuhr M, et al. Arthroscopic anatomy of the posterior ankle ligaments. Arthroscopy 2002;18(4):353–8.
19. Golanó P, Vega J, de Leeuw PA, et al. Anatomy of the ankle ligaments: a pictorial essay. Knee Surg Sports Traumatol Arthrosc 2010;18:557–69.
20. Rosenberg ZS, Cheung YY, Beltran J, et al. Posterior intermalleolar ligament of the ankle: normal anatomy and MR imaging features. AJR Am J Roentgenol 1995;165:387–90.
21. Milner CE, Soames RW. Anatomy of the collateral ligaments of the human ankle joint. Foot Ankle Int 1998;19:757–60.
22. Hamilton WG, Gepper MJ, Thompson FM. Pain in the posterior aspect of the ankle in dancers. Differential diagnosis and operative treatment. J Bone Joint Surg Am 1996;78:1491–500.
23. Oh CS, Won HS, Chung IH, et al. Anatomic variations and MRI of intermalleolar ligament. AJR Am J Roentgenol 2006;186:943–7.
24. Ugurlu M, Bozkurt M, Demirkale I, et al. Anatomy of the lateral complex of the ankle joint in relation to peroneal tendons, distal fibula and talus: a cadaveric study. Eklem Hastalik Cerrahisi 2010;21(3):153–8.
25. Panchani PN, Chappell TM, Moore GD, et al. Anatomic study of the deltoid ligament of the ankle. Foot Ankle Int 2014;35(9):916–21.
26. Cromeens BP, Kirchhoff CA, Patterson RM, et al. An attachment-based description of the medial collateral and spring ligament complexes. Foot Ankle Int 2015; 36(6):710–21.

Instrumentation in Arthroscopy

Eric A. Barp, DPM[a],*, John G. Erickson, DPM[b], Eric R. Reese, MS IV[c]

KEYWORDS

- Foot arthroscopy • Ankle arthroscopy • Arthroscopy instrumentation

KEY POINTS

- This article provides a basic understanding of the instrumentation typically used in foot and ankle arthroscopy.
- Arthroscopic instrumentation can be subdivided into 4 general categories: patient positioning, joint access, visualization, and debridement.
- It is important for surgeons to have a complete understanding of the instrumentation available to them, including indications and limitations.

INTRODUCTION

In recent years, arthroscopy has become popular in the treatment of many foot and ankle conditions. Many procedures have been found to be amenable to the arthroscopic approach, including, but not limited to, synovectomy, debridement, repair of osteochondral defects, evaluation of articular areas, arthrodesis procedures, and ligament repair. Although originally described for use in large articular areas, similar techniques have been described for other areas as well, including small joints, tendons, and bursae. Arthroscopy and endoscopy are now used to diagnose and treat conditions in many areas of the foot and ankle. This article introduces basic instrumentation used in foot and ankle arthroscopy.

The instruments used in arthroscopic surgery can be generally organized into 4 groups: patient positioning, access, visualization, and debridement.

PATIENT POSITIONING

Correct positioning of the patient before initiating the surgical procedure is crucial for the success of the planned procedure. Positioning may vary, depending on the type of arthroscopic procedure being performed and necessary portals; however, most procedures are performed with the patient in a supine position with the patient's feet even

[a] The Iowa Clinic, 5950 University Avenue, West Des Moines, IA 50266, USA; [b] UnityPoint Health, 1415 Woodland Avenue, Suite 100, Des Moines, IA 50309, USA; [c] Des Moines University, Des Moines, IA 50265, USA
* Corresponding author.
E-mail address: ebarp@iowaclinic.com

with the end of the operating table. An ipsilateral hip bump may be used to internally rotate the lower extremity to a rectus alignment. Positioning devices may also be used near the ankle to elevate the lower extremity off the table for easier instrument access and manipulation of the extremity. A thigh, or calf, tourniquet may also be used for hemostasis throughout the procedure; however, this is not a requirement (**Fig. 1**).

Techniques have also been described to ease the arthroscopy procedure and eliminate the need for distraction devices. Some surgeons find it easier to hang the knee over the edge of the table, allowing the leg to hang freely at 90°. This position allows access to all areas of the ankle joint and uses gravity to increase the articular space.[1]

Distraction in conjunction with a knee holder may also be used to increase visibility by widening the joint space. Many distraction techniques are available, and may be divided into invasive and noninvasive types.

Noninvasive distractors typically use an ankle strap with a distraction device attached to the operating table. Simple modifications have been described in the literature, including the use of a Kerlix gauze roll, as described by Yates and Grana.[2] Often these harnesses are attached to the surgeon's waist, which allows increased and decreased distraction by leaning forward or back. Although affordable and effective, it is difficult to gauge the amount of force being applied and patient harm may occur if excessive distraction is applied.

Invasive distraction is generally reserved for circumstances in which noninvasive attempts have failed, and its use is rarely required.[3] One style of invasive distraction, described by Guhl,[4] involves threaded pins placed through the tibia and calcaneus, then attached to a distraction device. This construct allows for distraction of up to 7 to 8 mm beyond normal joint space; however, it also introduces multiple potential complications.

De Leeuw and colleagues[5] found that distraction of the ankle joint places neurovascular structures at higher risk of damage as the stretch pulls the structures closer to the anterior aspect of the distal tibia. They also found that a slight dorsiflexory force of the ankle was more effective in protecting the neurovascular bundle because the laxity allowed increased distance between neurovascular structures and the distal portion of the anterior tibia, resulting in fewer complications and less risk of damage.

ACCESS

Arthroscopic portals are established through stab incisions through the skin and subcutaneous tissue with a number 11 scalpel blade. After the incision has been made, a cannula is inserted into the joint with the assistance of a sharp trocar or a blunt obturator. The cannula is a hollow stainless steel tube that is used to maintain a portal for access to the joint, protect the soft tissue from repeated insertion and removal of

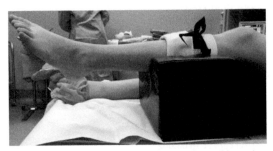

Fig. 1. Positioning device used to elevate the extremity for ankle arthroscopy.

instrumentation, and protect the fragile arthroscope. Many cannulas are equipped with valves that accept ingress or egress fluid systems (**Fig. 2**).

The cannula accepts the trocar and obturator for joint insertion. A trocar is a sharp instrument inserted into the cannula to pierce through the capsule. Caution must be taken with insertion of the trocar because of the sharp tip and blind insertion. If inserted too deeply this can cause damage to the cartilaginous surface of the joint. Obturators are round-tipped instruments inserted into the cannula allowing access to the joint without risk of damage to the cartilaginous surface. Once removed, the cannula is left in place, allowing entry of other instruments into the articular space. Other portals can be established to allow another location for insertion of the scope for visualization, or irrigation solution with an ingress/egress pump (**Fig. 3**).

Irrigation fluid, generally normal saline or lactated Ringer, helps control visualization of the arthroscopic field. Although irrigation with both solutions has been shown to cause acute stress to articular cartilage, neutral solutions such as lactated Ringer are recommended because of increased inhibition of normal production of proteoglycans by the chondrocytes with the use of saline.[6] Dilute epinephrine is also useful in arthroscopic surgery as a vasoconstrictor to decrease bleeding, resulting in increased visibility, shorter surgical times, and the need for less irrigation fluid.[7]

Typically, fluid ingress provided by gravity flow or pressure bags is sufficient to insufflate the joint; however, ingress-egress pumps are becoming more commonly used. Newer pumps are mechanically driven pressure systems with safety features such as high-pressure shut-downs and alarms for malfunctioning equipment. By controlling the flow rate, the surgeon can control the pressure and joint distention. A study by Ogilvie-Harris and Weisleder[8] showed decreased operative times, less soft tissue extravasation, better visibility, and better technical ease with ingress pumps that allow control of pressure and flow versus pumps that just control pressure. Although safety features are built into newer models, note that extravasation of fluid and even compartment syndrome are possible complications that need to be monitored closely.[9]

VISUALIZATION

The arthroscopy tower consists primarily of visualization instrumentation with the addition of the motorized power unit and occasionally an ingress-egress pump. This

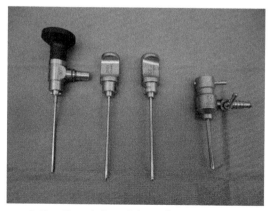

Fig. 2. Access instrumentation. From left to right: arthroscope, sharp trocar, blunt obturator, and cannula with an ingress valve.

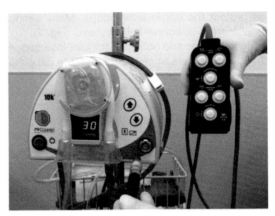

Fig. 3. Ingress pump with safety features.

organizational structure assists operating room staff to efficiently transition between patients. The chain of visualization starts with the arthroscopic camera, the progresses to a media control panel, and then to a high-definition monitor. The light source is an important component of the visualization instrumentation as well, and is connected to the camera by means of a fiberoptic cable. Recent improvements in digital image capture systems have greatly improved arthroscopic capabilities and have largely replaced older still photograph and video documentation. Most modern arthroscopy towers are also equipped with some form of digital media output such as DVD writers, USB drives, or printers. This equipment allows images to easily be recorded, edited, printed, or saved with ease, providing documentation of the procedure for medical records or patient education.

Continuous illumination of the arthroscope is provided by a fiberoptic cable from a light source. Cable length should be enough to reach the sterile field from the power unit, but not so long that it is difficult to control and risks contamination of the sterile field. Light sources have evolved over the years and currently many different types are available, including xenon arc lamps, tungsten illumination, mercury vapor lamps, and more recently LED (light-emitting diode) light sources. Xenon bulbs are generally considered the best option for arthroscopy because of their ability to provide better color quality. However, these bulbs are also expensive and need to be replaced every 500 to 600 hours at a cost of $400 to $700. Cold light sources, such as LED lights, come with much longer operating times (some >20,000 hours), but have lower power output. New imaging systems are capable of automatically adjusting light intensity to improve visibility.

It is also important to note that hot light sources, such as xenon bulbs, transmit heat to the articular areas, which can warm fluid and tissues, resulting in cellular damage and even death. Multiple studies have shown the effects of different temperature solutions, showing that fluid temperatures consistent with normal joint temperatures are most physiologic and least likely to cause damage (**Fig. 4**).[10,11]

The incorporation of video has greatly improved arthroscopic capabilities compared with initial arthroscopy, which was performed by direct visualization through an eyepiece. Newer technology allows projection of the image onto high-definition video screens. This technology has reduced the risk of contamination and improved depth perception and the surgeon's ability to make fine movements, as well as increasing the comfort of the surgeon. At present, arthroscopic lenses are available in different sizes

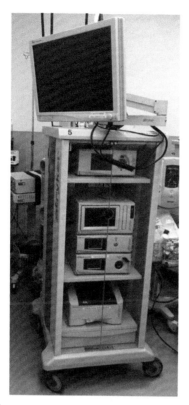

Fig. 4. Arthroscopic tower.

and fields of view. The most commonly used scopes are 1.9 mm, 2.7 mm, and 4.0 mm in diameter. Each of these scopes has a set viewing angle; most commonly a 30° or 70° scope is used. Smaller diameter scopes allow the instrumentation to be maneuvered into tights spaces; however, they are also structurally weaker and therefore more likely to be damaged within the joint space. Larger scopes also allow more room to house optical lenses and light-carrying fiberoptics, have increased irrigation abilities, and provide a larger field of view. Although the 30° scopes are most common and are adequate for the treatment of most disorders, the 70° scope can allow the surgeon to visualize the posterior ankle or within the ankle gutters with greater ease (**Fig. 5**).[12]

DEBRIDEMENT

A multitude of instruments are in production that are in the debridement category. These instruments are specially designed to provide treatment through minimal incisions and arthroscopic visualization. Curettes, osteotomes, forceps, graspers, probes, microfracture picks, powered shavers, burrs, and bone cutters are just a few of these instruments (**Fig. 6**).

Basket forceps are biting instruments used for cutting soft tissue such as loose fibrocartilage bodies. These forceps are available in straight or angled versions to increase maneuverability in small joint arthroscopy (**Fig. 7**).

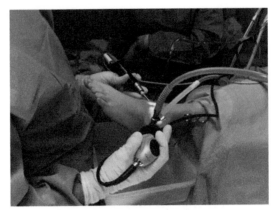

Fig. 5. Typical patient positioning with arthroscope and shaver introduced through standard anterior portals.

Grasping forceps are not cutting instruments but are used to firmly grasp bone fragments or loose bodies and remove them from the joint space (**Fig. 8**).

Osteotomes are chisel-like tools used for resecting bone. Like the other instruments discussed, osteotomes are also available in many shapes and orientations for increased accessibility in small joints. Elevators may also be used for similar purposes.

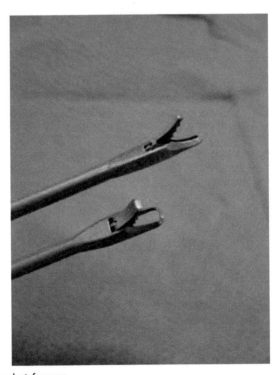

Fig. 6. Straight basket forceps.

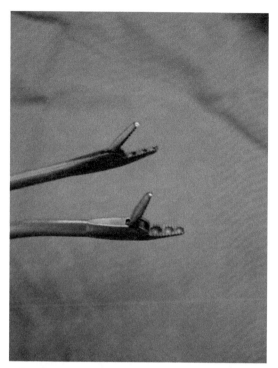

Fig. 7. Straight grasping forceps.

Electrocautery and arthroscopic ablators are also useful tools in arthroscopic surgery. They can be used for tissue dissection, soft tissue debridement, and coagulation to control bleeding. However, care must be taken when using cautery, because damage to the surrounding tissues is possible,[13] especially when using bipolar devices.[14] Studies have shown an increase in fluid temperature of the joint with the use of cautery, which furthers joint damage. Maintaining fluid flow with the use of ingress pumps

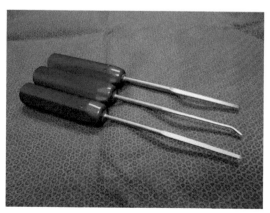

Fig. 8. Osteotomes.

has proved helpful in controlling the temperature and minimizing the risks associated with electrocautery (**Fig. 9**).

Probes function as an extension of the surgeon's fingers and are necessary for diagnostic arthroscopy. They can be used to palpate structures, determine consistency, determine depth, and maneuver intraarticular structures for improved visibility. Probes are among the most important tools used for arthroscopic surgery. They vary in size, length, and shape for ease of grasping the instrument and manipulating it in small articular spaces (**Fig. 10**).

Microfracture picks are available in many different sizes and angled tips designed specifically for use in small joint arthroscopy. These picks are used in articular cartilage repair to create small fractures, facilitating the formation of fibrocartilage. Traditional picks are tapped with a mallet to create the microfracture; however, electrically powered picks are now also being used (**Fig. 11**).

Ring curettes are available in a wide variety of shapes and sizes. These tools are used for bone resection or remodeling articular cartilage margins after the removal of an osteochondral defect.

Spoon curettes can also be used for debridement of osteochondral defects or subchondral bone cysts. Rasps or files may be used to smooth areas following debridement with curettes (**Fig. 12**).

Vector guides can be used for precise placement of guidewires and cannulated screws during small joint arthroscopic procedures. These devices are commonly described for use in repair of osteochondral defects, fracture stabilization, and internal fixation of fractures or arthrodesis (**Fig. 13**).

Power attachments such as motorized abraders, burrs, or shavers are very effective tools and allow increased efficiency in arthroscopic surgery. These instruments consist of an outer hollow metal sheath and an inner rotating blade or burr, and are run by a motorized rotary power unit that sits outside the sterile field. Motorized tools are easily controlled by buttons on the handpiece or a foot pedal. These tools can be run at variable speeds and are often connected to a suction device to remove debris from the joint space, allowing better visibility. Heat injuries to both tissue and equipment can also result when joint spaces are not irrigated adequately. Shavers use suction to draw tissue into the shaver, where it can be cut by the rotating blade. Larger cutting windows and different blade edges allow more aggressive debridement.

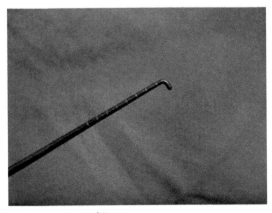

Fig. 9. Probe with measurement markings.

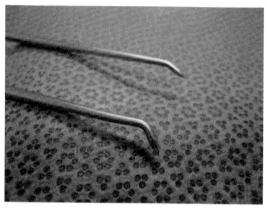

Fig. 10. Microfracture picks.

Suction force can be controlled to prevent aggressive movement of the tissue or turbulence of joint fluid, which may decrease visibility (**Fig. 14**).

Shaver speed is also an important factor with motorized equipment. Bone shavers, which typically have large blades and a large space between blades, are typically run at high speeds to prevent the shaver from jumping and damaging tissue. Soft tissue is better debrided at slower speeds, because these speeds allow more time for tissue to enter the open window and be cut by the blade.

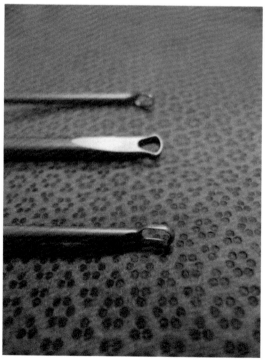

Fig. 11. Ring curettes.

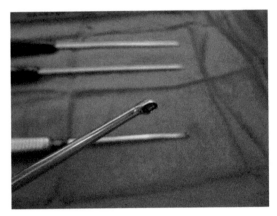

Fig. 12. Spoon curette.

STERILIZATION OF EQUIPMENT

Although the metal instruments can easily be autoclaved, steam autoclave has been sparsely used for motorized equipment because of heavy wear and tear placed on the delicate arthroscopy equipment, especially on seals, adhesives, and other plastics. Another option used for cleaning is a 2% glutaraldehyde disinfectant solution, which was thought to result in minimal infection rates and less damage to arthroscopy equipment,[15] but was later linked to a series of gas gangrene infections.[16] Some facilities have identified outbreaks following reuse of sterilized arthroscopy equipment, noting the probable cause to be retained tissue in the cannula and shaver pieces, allowing bacteria to survive.[17] Most equipment on the market currently is single use only, reducing the risk of dull blades or spread of infection or disease.

SUMMARY

In recent years, arthroscopic procedures of the foot and ankle have seen a significant increase in both indications and popularity. Furthermore, technological advances in video quality, fluid management, and other arthroscopy-specific instruments continue

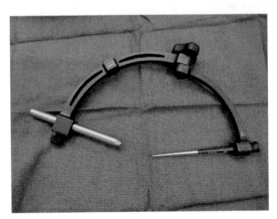

Fig. 13. Vector guide.

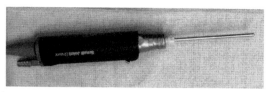

Fig. 14. Motorized arthroscopic shaver.

to make arthroscopic procedures more effective with reproducible outcomes. As surgeons continue to use this approach, it is important that they have a complete understanding of the instrumentation available to them, including their indications and limitations.

REFERENCES

1. Sun YQ, Slesarenko YA. Joint distraction may be unnecessary in ankle arthroscopy. Orthopedics 2006;29(2):118–20.
2. Yates CK, Grana WA. A simple distraction technique for ankle arthroscopy. Oklahoma City (OK): Oklahoma Center for Athletes; Orthopaedic Surgery and Rehabilitation; University of Oklahoma College of Medicine; 2006.
3. Palladino SJ. Distraction systems for ankle arthroscopy. Clin Podiatr Med Surg 1994;11:499–511.
4. Guhl JF. New concepts (distraction) in ankle arthroscopy. Milwaukee (WI): St Francis Hospital; Medical College of Wisconsin; 2006.
5. de Leeuw PA, Golano P, Clavero JA, et al. Anterior ankle arthroscopy, distraction or dorsiflexion? Knee Surg Sports Traumatol Arthrosc 2010;18:594–600.
6. Gulihar A, Bryson DJ, Taylor GJ. Effect of different irrigation fluids on human articular cartilage: an in vitro study. Arthroscopy 2013;29:251–6.
7. van Montfoort DO, van Kampen PM, Huijsmans PE. Epinephrine diluted saline-irrigation fluid in arthroscopic shoulder surgery: a significant improvement of clarity of visual field and shortening of total operation time. a randomized controlled trial. Arthroscopy 2016;32(3):436–44.
8. Ogilvie-Harris DJ, Weisleder L. Fluid pump systems for arthroscopy: a comparison of pressure control versus pressure and flow control. Arthroscopy 1995;11:591–5.
9. Bomberg BC, Hurley PE, Clark CA, et al. Complications associated with the use of an infusion pump during knee arthroscopy. Arthroscopy 1992;8(2):224–8.
10. Cheng SC, Jou IM, Chern TC, et al. The effect of normal saline irrigation at different temperatures on the surface of articular cartilage: an experimental study in the rat. Arthroscopy 2004;20:55–61.
11. Kocaoglu B, Martin J, Wolf B, et al. The effect of irrigation solution at different temperatures on articular cartilage metabolism. Arthroscopy 2011;27(4):526–31.
12. Spennacchio P, Randelli P, Arrigoni P, et al. Improved visualization of the 70° arthroscope in the treatment of talar osteochondral defects. Arthrosc Tech 2013;2(2):e129–33.
13. Lu Y, Edwards RB 3rd, Nho S, et al. Thermal chondroplasty with bipolar and monopolar radiofrequency energy: effect of treatment time on chondrocyte death and surface contouring. Arthroscopy 2002;18(7):779–88.
14. Edwards RB 3rd, Lu Y, Nho S, et al. Thermal chondroplasty of chondromalacic human cartilage. An ex vivo comparison of bipolar and monopolar radiofrequency devices. Am J Sports Med 2002;30(1):90–7.

15. Johnson LL, Shneider DA, Austin MD, et al. Two per cent glutaraldehyde: a disinfectant in arthroscopy and arthroscopic surgery. J Bone Joint Surg Am 1982; 64(2):237–9.
16. Herzberg W. Problems with the sterilisation and the maintenance of sterility of arthroscopic instruments: a comparison of different types of camera drapes. Knee Surg Sports Traumatol Arthrosc 1993;1(3–4):223–5.
17. Tosh PK, Disbot M, Duffy JM, et al. Outbreak of *Pseudomonas aeruginosa* surgical site infections after arthroscopic procedures: Texas, 2009. Infect Control Hosp Epidemiol 2011;32:1179–86.

Imaging of Common Arthroscopic Pathology of the Ankle

Sean T. Grambart, DPM

KEYWORDS

- Anterolateral ankle impingement • Anteromedial ankle impingement • Os trigonum
- Osteochondral lesion talus

KEY POINTS

- CT scan may be more beneficial in prognosis of osteochondral lesions.
- MRI seems to be the gold standard for imaging of impingement syndromes.
- Inflammation of the flexor hallucis longus tendon on MRI does not indicate os trigonum syndrome.

INTRODUCTION

Arthroscopy of the ankle is used in the treatment and diagnosis of a spectrum of intra-articular pathology, such as soft tissue and osseous impingement, osteochondral lesions, arthrofibrosis, and synovitis. To help identify the correct pathology, imaging techniques are often used to aid the surgeon in diagnosing pathology and determining best treatment options.

ANTEROLATERAL ANKLE IMPINGEMENT

Routine radiographs may show spurring along the anterior ankle joint line on the lateral view, but this view cannot confirm exact location of the spur. Gold standard imaging is an MRI. However, controversy occurs as to how accurate MRI is for the identification of impingement syndrome. Ferkel and colleagues[1] studied 31 patients with more than 2 years of follow-up who had chronic anterolateral ankle pain following inversion injury. All had failed to respond to at least 2 months of conservative treatment and had negative stress radiographs to rule out instability. On physical examination, tenderness was localized to the anterolateral corner of the talar dome. MRI was the most useful diagnostic screening test, showing synovial thickening consistent with impingement in the anterolateral gutter.

Liu and colleagues[2] reviewed 22 patients who had arthroscopic evaluations and preoperative MRI studies of their ankles because of chronic anterolateral ankle pain

Carle Physician Group, Department of Orthopedics, 1802 South Mattis Avenue, Champaign, IL 61821, USA
E-mail address: Sean.Grambart@Carle.com

Clin Podiatr Med Surg 33 (2016) 493–502
http://dx.doi.org/10.1016/j.cpm.2016.06.007   podiatric.theclinics.com
0891-8422/16/$ – see front matter © 2016 Elsevier Inc. All rights reserved.

after sprains. They tested the ability of surgeons to use the initial clinical examination to predict arthroscopically confirmed anterolateral ankle impingement compared with the ability to predict this condition using preoperative MRI. The patient population consisted of 15 men and 7 women who had an average age of 28 years. Five patients (23%) were intercollegiate athletes and 17 patients (77%) were recreational athletes. All patients reported previous trauma to the involved ankles, and all were seen with chronic ankle pain. Clinical examinations were used to assess ankle pain, swelling, range of motion, and stability. Anterolateral ankle impingement was confirmed in 18 patients (82%) with arthroscopic examination. Clinical examinations had a sensitivity of 94% and a specificity of 75% for predicting impingement, and MRI had a sensitivity of 39% and a specificity of 50%. The results of this study suggest that preoperative MRI examination is not beneficial or cost-effective in the diagnosis of anterolateral ankle impingement; furthermore, its use may cause further delay in treatment.

The use of intravenous contrast has been presented to try and enhance the soft tissue impingement. Bagnolesi and colleagues[3] reported mild to moderate contrast enhancement of the abnormal synovium in 8 of 14 patients with synovial impingement lesions. In patients with a mature meniscoid lesion, the hyalinized fibrosis is avascular and may not enhance. This situation may account for a recent study that found indirect MRI arthrography to be less accurate than conventional MRI of the ankle for diagnosis of impingement lesions.[4]

There have been several reports on the use of ultrasound to assess anterolateral ankle impingement. Cochet and colleagues[5] proposed ultrasound diagnostic criteria for synovial thickening along the anterolateral gutter of the ankle. Using these criteria, sensitivity, specificity, and accuracy of sonography in the diagnosis of anterolateral ankle impingement were 76%, 57%, and 73%, respectively. McCarthy and co-workers[6] described 10 patients with anterolateral impingement who had posttraumatic synovitis detected at ultrasound and later confirmed with arthroscopy. Hyperemia was not shown in the area of synovial thickening in any of their 10 patients. The investigators proposed a 10-mm cutoff size for the synovial thickening and the presence of anterolateral impingement symptoms.[6]

In anterolateral soft tissue impingement, MRI may show posttraumatic synovitis within the anterolateral gutter, which manifests as filiform intermediate signal intensity foci on proton density-weighted and fat-suppressed proton density-weighted or T2-weighted MRI sequences (**Fig. 1**).

Evaluation of the adjacent anterior talofibular and anterior-inferior tibiofibular ligaments can assess for evidence of previous injury. As the synovitis becomes more organized and undergoes hyalinized fibrosis, it appears confluent and progressively decreases in signal intensity. After arthroscopy, postsurgical scarring of the anterior lateral gutter capsule can mimic a meniscoid lesion on MRI. Clinically, however, this scarring is rarely symptomatic. Arthrofibrosis is visualized as anterior capsular thickening (>3 mm), which may be of intermediate signal on proton density-weighted MRI in the early phase, and become progressively lower in signal intensity over time. This shows up as a dense gray tissue on T1-weighted images (**Fig. 2**). In the early stages, there may be adjacent bone marrow edema in the anterior margin of the tibial plafond at the insertion of the anterior capsule.[7–9]

ANTEROMEDIAL ANKLE IMPINGEMENT

Anteromedial impingement spurs are best shown on an oblique radiograph of the foot. This projection involves a 45° craniocaudal angulation of the radiograph tube, with the leg positioned in 30° of external rotation.[10] Ultrasonography may show synovitis, scar,

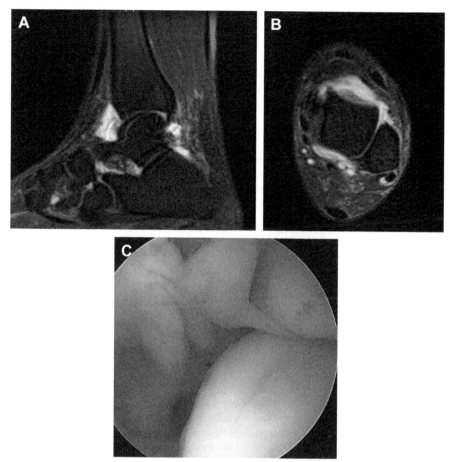

Fig. 1. Anterolateral impingement. (*A*) T2 sagittal MRI view of impingement. (*B*) T2 axial MRI view of impingement. (*C*) Arthroscopic visualization of impingement.

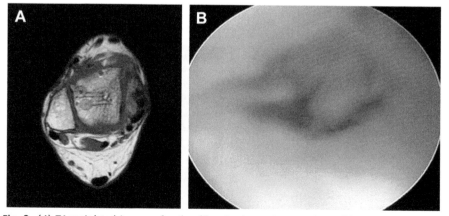

Fig. 2. (*A*) T1-weighted image of arthrofibrosis along the anterior ankle joint. (*B*) Arthroscopic findings consistent with arthrofibrosis. Dense, chronic synovial tissue.

and loose bodies in the anteromedial gutter. Computed tomography (CT) readily shows the location of any anteromedial ankle impingement spurs.

Initial reports of anteromedial impingement in the surgical literature suggested that MRI had been unhelpful in cases that had been diagnosed at surgery.[11] It has been reported that MRI arthrography may improve the conspicuity of medial meniscoid lesions, thickening of the anterior tibiotalar ligament, anteromedial capsular thickening, synovitis, bony spurs, and chondral or osteochondral lesions; however, it is a technique that is not widely used.[12]

MRI findings in anteromedial impingement with symptomatic spurs may include bone marrow edema within the spur and adjacent synovitis or capsular thickening in the anteromedial gutter and pericapsular edema (**Fig. 3**). Thickening and edema of the anterior tibiotalar ligament may be visualized in the sagittal and sometimes the coronal planes. Axial and sagittal images may show synovitis and fibrous bands in the anteromedial gutter.[9]

POSTERIOR ANKLE IMPINGEMENT

Standard foot radiographs may be used to identify an os trigonum or a Stieda process. An os trigonum may be superimposed on the posterolateral process of the talus on a straight lateral projection (**Fig. 4**). Augmentation of a routine ankle series with a lazy lateral view where the ankle is mildly externally rotated, and a lateral view in plantar flexion can help show an os trigonum that remains occult on a standard lateral view and may show bony abutment in plantar flexion.[9]

Ultrasonography may be a useful technique for the assessment and management of posterior impingement.[13] Injections for posterior impingement associated with an os trigonum may be performed under ultrasound or fluoroscopic guidance. Injections of this nature may be diagnostic and therapeutic.[14,15]

The MRI protocol used for investigating posterior ankle impingement should adequately show a small os trigonum, myxoid change in the posterior talofibular ligament, posterior ankle ganglia, flexor hallucis longus (FHL) tendon disease, and synovitis. The protocols vary according to the MRI unit and personal preference. Recommendations should include sagittal and axial proton density-weighted and fat-suppressed proton density-weighted, and coronal proton density-weighted sequences in the study.[9]

The size of an os trigonum or degree of prominence of the posterolateral process of the talus is not strongly correlated with the severity of posterior impingement symptoms.[16]

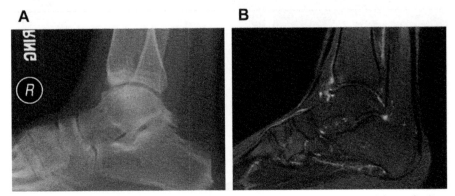

Fig. 3. (*A*) Radiographic view of anteromedial ankle osseous impingement. (*B*) MRI findings consistent with soft tissue anterior impingement.

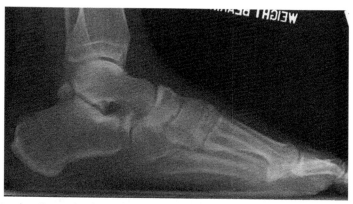

Fig. 4. Lateral radiograph of prominent os trigonum.

Changes seen using ultrasound include myxoid change in the posterior talofibular ligament and complicating ganglion cyst formation in some patients with posterior impingement.[9]

CT is able to characterize pathologic changes at the interface between the os trigonum and talus, including cystic change and sclerosis at the synchondrosis margins and widening of the synchondrosis (**Fig. 5**).[17]

MRI findings have the value of evaluating the bone and the tendon. On T1-weighted or proton density-weighted sequences, an os trigonum usually shows fatty marrow signal intensity and corticated margins. Bone marrow edema within the os may occur in active posterior impingement (**Fig. 6**). Sclerosis within the os is less common. Occasionally, pericapsular fat may mimic an os trigonum. Conventional MRI can accurately identify disease at the synchondrosis. Signal hyperintensity at the synchondrosis on proton density-weighted or T2-weighted MRI with fat suppression usually indicates a degree of stress across the synchondrosis and is often associated with bone marrow edema at the synchondrosis margins. Frank fluid signal at the synchondrosis indicates destabilization. Findings that are likely to be associated with posterior ankle impingement symptoms include bone marrow edema at the margins of the synchondrosis, synovitis involving the posterior recesses of the ankle and posterior subtalar joint, and pericapsular edema and increased fluid within the flexor hallucis longus

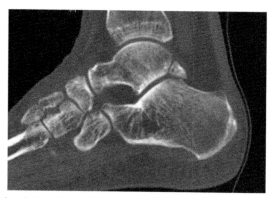

Fig. 5. CT scan with subchondral cystic changes of the os trigonum.

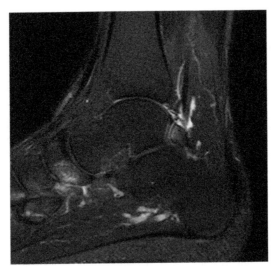

Fig. 6. MRI finding with increased signal intensity consistent with bone marrow edema along the os trigonum.

tendon sheath. Sclerosis and cystic change at the margins of the synchondrosis indicate chronic stress across the synchondrosis. Bone marrow edema may be seen in a prominent posterolateral talar process in the setting of active posterior impingement.[7,9]

Sagittal MRIs are used to assess the posterolateral process of the talus. The posterolateral process is considered prominent if it extends posterior to the arc of curvature of the talar dome in the sagittal plane. Recent fractures of the posterolateral process show bone marrow edema and linear T1 hypointensity at the fracture line.[9]

FHL tendon disease may mimic or accompany posterior impingement symptoms. MRI is of limited sensitivity for the diagnosis of FHL tendinosis.[7] Fluid distention of the FHL tendon sheath can also be present in asymptomatic ankles. An FHL tendon sheath effusion in the absence of an ankle or posterior subtalar joint effusion is more suggestive of FHL tenosynovitis, but is still nonspecific.

OSTEOCHONDRAL LESIONS

Initial imaging is standard weightbearing ankle radiographs. Osteochondral fractures or osteochondral defects (OCD) lesions are not always visualized on plain films, particularly stage I Berndt and Hardy lesions.[18] These occult lesions are usually seen on MRI. Radiographs that visualize osteochondral lesions usual indicate cystic changes within the bone (**Fig. 7**).

MRI is more frequently used in the diagnosis and staging of OCD lesions of the talus and is valuable in aiding in the diagnosis of adjacent tissue injuries and the osteochondral lesion. This imaging modality can evaluate breaches in the articular cartilage, signal intensity changes of the subchondral bone, and loose bodies in the ankle joint (**Fig. 8**).[19–21] Other important factors including peroneal tendon tears, characteristics of the osteochondral lesions, can sometimes be clearly identified by MRI.

Verhagen and colleagues[22] summarized all eligible studies to compare the effectiveness of different treatment strategies for OCD of the talus. They looked at 39 studies describing the results of treatment strategies for OCD of the talus. When

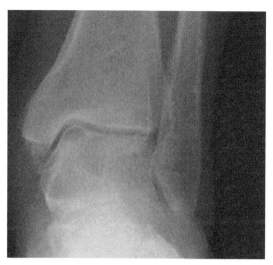

Fig. 7. Anteroposterior radiograph of the ankle showing cystic changes of the osteochondral lesion along the medial talus.

identifying and evaluating osteochondral lesions they found diagnostic arthroscopy demonstrated a sensitivity of 1 and specificity of 0.97. MRI without contrast resulted in 0.96 sensitivity and specificity. CT scans had a sensitivity and specificity of 0.81 and 0.99. Mortise view radiographs demonstrated sensitivity and specificity of 0.7 and

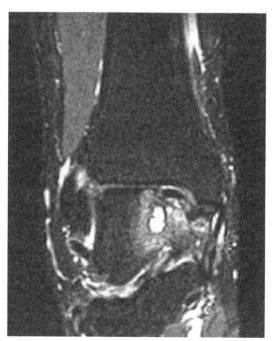

Fig. 8. MRI with increased signal intensity, cystic changes, and articular damage in osteochondral lesion.

0.94, whereas history and physical examination was least sensitive (0.59) and specific (0.91).

CT scans have shown that lesions are larger than appreciated on radiograph, and CT scan is useful in preoperative planning by determining the size and depth of OCD lesions.[23–25]

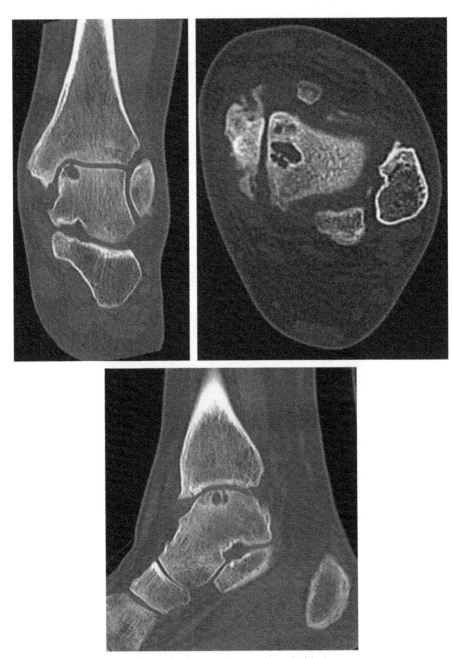

Fig. 9. CT scans showing the cystic changes in osteochondral lesion.

Nakasa and colleagues[26] evaluated the relationship between arthroscopic findings and CT scan of osteochondral lesions. Patients underwent CT, MRI, and arthroscopic surgery. The three types for cystic lesion ankles were irregular shape, round shape with sclerotic wall, and irregular shape with opening to an articular cavity. The three types for fragment lesion were no bone absorption, bed absorption without fragment absorption, and bed sclerosis and fragment absorption. Results showed all round and sclerotic cystic lesions revealed cartilaginous flap lesions with a nearly normal cartilage surface. An irregular shape with opening revealed an unstable lesion with severely damaged cartilage. Regarding fragment lesions, no absorption revealed a stable lesion with a nearly normal cartilage surface. Bed absorption revealed an unstable lesion with a nearly normal cartilage surface. Fragment absorption with bed sclerosis showed an unstable lesion with severely damaged cartilage. There was a significant difference between CT findings and International Cartilage Repair Society grade or arthroscopic findings (both $P<.01$), whereas there was no significant difference with MRI grading. The diagnosis of cartilage status by CT was better than MRI.

The author typically recommends beginning with an MRI to evaluate the osteochondral lesion and adjacent pathology. However, in large lesions with osseous changes, the author obtains a CT scan to accurately assess the adjacent bone to help determine size and the best treatment options (**Fig. 9**).

REFERENCES

1. Ferkel RD, Karzel RP, Del Pizzo W, et al. Arthroscopic treatment of anterolateral impingement of the ankle. Am J Sports Med 1991;19(5):440–6.

2. Liu SH, Nuccion SL, Finerman G. Diagnosis of anterolateral ankle impingement. Comparison between magnetic resonance imaging and clinical examination. Am J Sports Med 1997;25(3):389–93.

3. Bagnolesi P, Zampa V, Carafoli D, et al. Anterolateral fibrous impingement of the ankle. Report of 14 cases. Radiol Med 1998;95(4):293–7 [in Italian].

4. Haller J, Bernt R, Seeger T, et al. MR-imaging of anterior tibiotalar impingement syndrome: agreement, sensitivity and specificity of MR-imaging and indirect MR-arthrography. Eur J Radiol 2006;58(3):450–60.

5. Cochet H, Pelé E, Amoretti N, et al. Anterolateral ankle impingement: diagnostic performance of MDCT arthrography and sonography. AJR Am J Roentgenol 2010;194(6):1575–80.

6. McCarthy CL, Wilson DJ, Coltman TP. Anterolateral ankle impingement: findings and diagnostic accuracy with ultrasound imaging. Skeletal Radiol 2008;37(3):209–16.

7. Linklater J. MR imaging of ankle impingement lesions. Magn Reson Imaging Clin N Am 2009;17(4):775–800, vii–viii.

8. Linklater JM, Fessa CK. Imaging findings in arthrofibrosis of the ankle and foot. Semin Musculoskelet Radiol 2012;16(3):185–91.

9. Dimmick S, Linklater J. Ankle impingement syndromes. Radiol Clin North Am 2013;51(3):479–510.

10. van Dijk CN, Wessel RN, Tol JL, et al. Oblique radiograph for the detection of bone spurs in anterior ankle impingement. Skeletal Radiol 2002;31(4):214–21.

11. Mosier-La Clair SM, Monroe MT, Manoli A. Medial impingement syndrome of the anterior tibiotalar fascicle of the deltoid ligament on the talus. Foot Ankle Int 2000; 21(5):385–91.

12. Robinson P, White LM, Salonen D, et al. Anteromedial impingement of the ankle: using MR arthrography to assess the anteromedial recess. AJR Am J Roentgenol 2002;178(3):601–4.
13. Robinson P. Impingement syndromes of the ankle. Eur Radiol 2007;17(12): 3056–65.
14. Jaffee NW, Gilula LA, Wissman RD, et al. Diagnostic and therapeutic ankle tenography: outcomes and complications. AJR Am J Roentgenol 2001;176(2):365–71.
15. Mouhsine E, Crevoisier X, Leyvraz PF, et al. Post-traumatic overload or acute syndrome of the os trigonum: a possible cause of posterior ankle impingement. Knee Surg Sports Traumatol Arthrosc 2004;12(3):250–3.
16. Hamilton WG, Geppert MJ, Thompson FM. Pain in the posterior aspect of the ankle in dancers. Differential diagnosis and operative treatment. J Bone Joint Surg Am 1996;78(10):1491–500.
17. Karasick D, Schweitzer ME. The os trigonum syndrome: imaging features. AJR Am J Roentgenol 1996;166(1):125–9.
18. O'Farrell TA, Costello BG. Osteochondritis dissecans of the talus. The late results of surgical treatment. J Bone Joint Surg Br 1982;64(4):494–7.
19. De Smet AA, Fisher DR, Burnstein MI, et al. Value of MR imaging in staging osteochondral lesions of the talus (osteochondritis dissecans): results in 14 patients. AJR Am J Roentgenol 1990;154(3):555–8.
20. Nelson DW, DiPaola J, Colville M, et al. Osteochondritis dissecans of the talus and knee: prospective comparison of MR and arthroscopic classifications. J Comput Assist Tomogr 1990;14(5):804–8.
21. Talusan PG, Milewski MD, Toy JO, et al. Osteochondritis dissecans of the talus: diagnosis and treatment in athletes. Clin Sports Med 2014;33(2):267–84.
22. Verhagen RA, Struijs PA, Bossuyt PM, et al. Systematic review of treatment strategies for osteochondral defects of the talar dome. Foot Ankle Clin 2003;8(2): 233–42, viii–ix.
23. Davies AM, Cassar-Pullicino VN. Demonstration of osteochondritis dissecans of the talus by coronal computed tomographic arthrography. Br J Radiol 1989; 62(744):1050–5.
24. Higuera J, Laguna R, Peral M, et al. Osteochondritis dissecans of the talus during childhood and adolescence. J Pediatr Orthop 1998;18(3):328–32.
25. Zinman C, Wolfson N, Reis ND. Osteochondritis dissecans of the dome of the talus. Computed tomography scanning in diagnosis and follow-up. J Bone Joint Surg Am 1988;70(7):1017–9.
26. Nakasa T, Adachi N, Kato T, et al. Correlation between subchondral bone plate thickness and cartilage degeneration in osteoarthritis of the ankle. Foot Ankle Int 2014;35(12):1341–9.

Soft Tissue Impingement of the Ankle

Pathophysiology, Evaluation, and Arthroscopic Treatment

Amber M. Shane, DPM, FACFAS*, Christopher L. Reeves, DPM, FACFAS, Ryan Vazales, DPM, Zachary Farley, DPM

KEYWORDS

- Ankle impingement • Anterolateral ankle impingement • Synovitis • Meniscoid body
- Ankle pain

KEY POINTS

- Chronic soft tissue impingement of the tibiotalar joint often begins with an inciting injury involving a severe inversion-plantar flexion or eversion-dorsiflexion biomechanical pathway.
- Understanding the mechanism of action responsible for primary pathology and completing a strong medical history is paramount to the clinician identifying the correct diagnosis.
- Loss of either the lateral or medial ligamentous structures responsible for stability of the ankle joint can lead to uncoupling of the foot and tibia ending in gross instability and chronic pain. These types of ankle injuries are often poly-traumatic, and prompt identification and adequate time for healing is required for consistent good long-term results.
- Soft tissue impingement of the ankle should be suspected in any patients who present with a chief complaint of chronic pain secondary to an injury or sprain.
- When conservative treatment options fail, arthroscopy as a monotherapy, and sometimes combined with open resection of this pathology, is an effective treatment paradigm that has produced good to excellent long-term results.

INTRODUCTION

Soft tissue impingement (STI) syndrome is one of 3 causes of a larger all-encompassing joint impingement pathology, which includes bone and neuropathic entrapment as well.[1] It has been described in the literature for multiple joint surfaces

Reconstructive Foot and Ankle Surgery, Orlando Foot and Ankle Clinic, 250 North Alafaya Trail, Suite 115, Orlando, FL 32825, USA
* Corresponding author.
E-mail address: ashane@orlandofootandankle.com

Clin Podiatr Med Surg 33 (2016) 503–520
http://dx.doi.org/10.1016/j.cpm.2016.06.003
0891-8422/16/© 2016 Elsevier Inc. All rights reserved.

within the body. Altered joint biomechanics and friction of joint tissues combine to cause chronic pain and often functional instability. Regarding arthroscopic treatment of STI in the lower extremity, much of the literature has been centered on athletes and the tibiotalar joint, in particular anterior ankle impingement. Originally described by Morris[2] in his report of athletes ankle in 1943, STI of the ankle joint now encompasses a combination of pathologies whereby anatomic structures surrounding the tibiotalar joint become entrapped leading to decreased range of motion (ROM) and often present as chronic pain syndrome clinically. Although the most common form of STI to the ankle is anterolateral in location, posterior and anteromedial impingement is also discussed in this article. Furthermore, a discussion of biomechanical deficiencies, that is, varus/valgus foot, and how they may effect location and cause of STI of the ankle is explored along with pathophysiology, clinical and diagnostic evaluation, current treatments, and long-term outcomes.

ANATOMY

Ankle sprains involving the ligamentous soft tissue structures of the ankle joint are most commonly seen in athletic injuries, with as much as 20% of them showing residual and even chronic pain symptoms.[3] Pathologic findings after ankle sprain injuries often include impingement lesions, peroneal tendinopathy, ligamentous laxity, boney sequela, and even osteochondral lesions.[4] Although most resolve with rest, ice, compression, elevation, and physical therapy, a study by Smith and Reischl[5] in 1986 revealed that 50% of the study population of basketball players showed residual clinical symptomology and 15% even noted decreased performance capabilities. Often times the extent and location of soft tissue pathology and painful tibiotalar instability is determined by foot position and the direction and magnitude of forces applied to the joint.

Two ligamentous complexes stabilize the tibiotalar joint. Laterally, the joint houses 3 ligamentous structures: the anteroinferior tibiofibular ligament (AITFL), the posteroinferior tibiofibular ligament (PITFL), and the interosseous tibiofibular ligament, which is a continuation of the interosseous membrane. This structure known as the lateral collateral ligament (LCL) complex of the ankle functions to allow the distal tibia and fibula to act as one unit when adapting to changes in ground reactive forces being applied. Medially, the deltoid ligament stabilizes the ankle joint with both superficial and deep attachments known as the medial collateral ligament (MCL) complex of the ankle. The superficial portion crosses 2 joints, including the ankle and subtalar joint, whereas the deep complex crosses only one and has been implicated in the cause of medial STI syndrome. The inferior lateral ligament complex (LLC) is composed of the anterior talofibular ligament (ATFL), calcaneofibular ligament, and the posterior talofibular ligament (PTFL); although it is not directly associated with the ankle mortise, it too has been implicated in the pathophysiology of ankle STI syndrome.

CAUSE

By far, the most common type of STI of the ankle joint is anterolateral in its location. Anterolateral STI (ALSTI) is implicated in approximately 3% of all ankle sprains and is associated with injuries involving both the LCL and LLC, which often occur because of a plantar flexion inversion mechanism.[6,7] It should be considered as a primary diagnoses in patients with long-standing ankle pain or functional ankle instability when bone and arthritic pathology have been ruled out. ALSTI encompasses 3 types of lesions: (1) meniscoid lesion (Wolin lesion), (2) synovitis, and (3) impingement of the AITFL distal fascicle (Bassett ligament).

Meniscoid lesions or Wolin lesion, so named for their similarity in appearance to that of the knee meniscus, were first described by Wolin and colleagues[8] in 1950. In their study of 9 patients who had sustained inversion ankle sprains and presented with chronic ankle pain, they described their surgical findings as soft tissue masses of hyalinized scar tissue associated with fibrous adhesions from the ATFL (**Fig. 1**). Although not true ligamentous tears, these adhesions were noted to extend into the lateral gutter of the ankle and cause pain with the ankle placed in maximum dorsiflexion for both active and passive ROM. This finding was further supported by Ferkel and colleagues[6] in 1991 who demonstrated histologically that the lesions associated with the ATFL were not ligamentous tears but rather fibrous bands of inflamed tissue and likely the cause of STI to the ankle.

Chronic synovitis has been described as inflammation with enlargement of the ligamentous ends of a ligament rupture and has been implicated as another cause of ALSTI of the ankle.[6] Often associated with a tear of the ATFL, the inflamed synovium is caused by inadequate immobilization and healing which leads to entrapment of tissues within the lateral gutter causing pain (**Fig. 2**). Furthermore, over time, chronic scar tissue formation and decreased dorsiflexory ROM ensues. Additionally, hypertrophied synovium within the lateral gutter of the ankle known as a "synovial shelf" can be present after inversion ankle sprains, which often extends over the anterior lateral superior portion of the talus and is associated with ALSTI.[9] This finding was similar to a "synovial Plicae" described previously by Amendola and colleagues.[10]

Torn capsulitis and/or rupture of the AITFL combined with inadequate healing, recurrent motion, and instability have been thought to be another underlying cause for ALSTI.[11] However, there have been multiple descriptions in the literature regarding an accessory and/or separate distal fascicle of the AITFL, which has been noted to play a role in primary ALSTI. Nikolopoulos'[12] study in 1982 (never published in English) was first to describe an "accessory AITFL," which they thought was a continuation of the AITFL. This idea of an "accessory ligament" was later challenged by Bassett and colleagues,[13] describing a completely separate distal fascicle of the AITF, noting a well-delineated fibrofatty septum separating the two ligaments.[13] The separate ligamentous fascicle was later coined *Bassett ligament* (see **Fig. 1**). Ray and Kriz[14] provided an anatomic description of the distal fascicle, also called Bassett ligament in

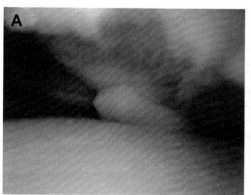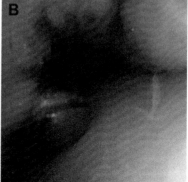

Fig. 1. Meniscoid Wolin lesion impinging the anterolateral gutter of the ankle joint (*A*). Arthroscopic debridement of meniscoid body with shaver device (*B*).

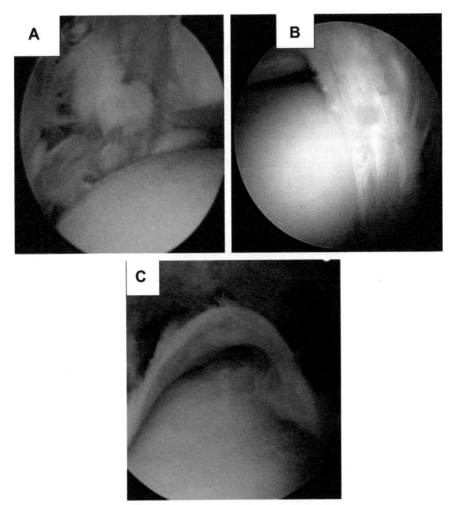

Fig. 2. Acute on chronic synovitis causing STI to the anterolateral ankle gutter (*A*). Image showing distal fascicle Bassett ligament with noted fraying of ligamentous edges (*B*). Meniscal or plicated synovial bodies (*C*).

their report of 46 specimens. Their findings showed 10 specimens had a ligament that was parallel and distal to the AITFL. The fibers traveled obliquely from the anterolateral distal aspect of the tibia to the anteromedial aspect of the fibula directly adjacent to the insertion of the ATFL. The fascicle measured 17 to 22 mm in length and 3 to 5 mm in width. Of note was that it crossed the anterolateral superior aspect of the talus.[14] The incidence differs very widely in multiple studies likely because of different definitions of what constitutes a separate delineation of fibers.[13,15]

The distal fascicle of the AITFL, and its proximity and/or contact with anterolateral superior aspect of the talus, is a normal anatomic finding in most cases. However, this fascicle can become pathologic secondary to changes in ankle joint mechanics and instability in the frontal plane after injury and cause chronic impingement pain in some cases (see **Fig. 2**).[16] There have been multiple theories associated with the distal fascicle and its role in STI of the ankle. Bassett and colleagues[13] discussed the pathomechanism of the distal fascicle noted in patients with a history of inversion sprains and chronic hyperlaxity secondary to an injured ATFL. Furthermore, they suggested that this pathology caused an anterior projection of the talar dome, which led to greater contact forces on the anterolateral superior aspect of the talus with dorsiflexion and eventual impingement of soft tissue in the ankle gutter.[13] Akseki and colleagues[15] postulated that the length and width of the distal fascicle may play a role in the amount of bending and contact forces on the talus that could occur in dorsiflexion-eversion ROM, suggesting that those that were thicker and longer had a greater chance to have increased forces applied to the talus and lead to impingement. Even more, they noted that there was a posterior shift of the anterior talus with dorsiflexion with the ATFL intact; however, that shift was not seen, and the distal fascicle remained in contact when the AFTL was transected and the ankle was placed in dorsiflexion.[14] Additionally, Johnson and Markolf[17] found that anteroposterior laxity to the ankle joint was significantly increased with sectioning of the ATFL, particularly when placed in dorsiflexion.

Although this contact may be normal in some cases, Nikolopoulos[12] showed that increased bending of the distal fascicle led to greater tension of the ligamentous bands when in dorsiflexion and were likely associated with impingement. Furthermore, abraded articular cartilage over the anterolateral superior region of the talus was noted in multiple studies, which they suggested could be associated with talar dome remodeling due to increased fascicle contact with impingement of the soft tissue.[13-15] Hyperlaxity of the ligamentous tissue is often visualized arthroscopically with patients with STI and is an indication to evaluate both the ATFL and distal fascicle of the AITFL pathology. It should also be noted that arthroscopic or open resection of the distal fascicle does not increase ankle joint instability, as the pathology is likely secondary to ATFL pathology, which leads to instability at the ankle.[13,18]

Posterior STI of the tibiotalar joint has been discussed much less in the literature compared with that of the anterolateral position more commonly identified. It has been well established in the arthroscopic literature that the PITFL houses both a superficial and deep component.[19] Of note, the deep component (deep transverse ligament) has direct contact with the talus, which is visualized with anterior arthroscopic portals and provides posterior stability inhibiting posterior talar translation during ROM.[20] Although this structure rarely has isolated pathology, trauma to the ligamentous tissue could lead to posterior translation of the talus and cause chronic pain or impingement. This complication could further be exacerbated if patients have boney pathology associated with it, such as a Stieda process fracture or a large os trigonum.

The PTFL is found in nearly a horizontal plane coursing from the medial surface of the lateral malleolus with its fibers coming in intimate contact with the posterolateral talus. It is designated intracapsular extrasynovial with some fibers attaching to the lateral aspect of the talus, whereas others extend and can reach the talar tuber and even the os trigonum if present. The ligament is thick and spans a large surface area that even encompasses the posterior aspect of the tibia where its fibers fuse with those of the PITFL (deep branch).[20] This portion of the ligament has been labeled the "tibial slip" as first described by Chen[21] in 1985 and has been implicated in the cause of posterior STI of the ankle.[22] Its presence in anatomic dissection has a large range likely being due to the small size of the ligament on average 2 to 3 mm in size.[20] The "tibial slip" of the PTFL runs obliquely in an upward direction and is taught during dorsiflexory and relaxed during platarflexory ROM owing to its role in impingement of the ankle with traumatic forced dorsiflexory movements. Rupture of the ligamentous structure as well as possible avulsion of the posterior talar process from which the ligament attaches pose possible pathology that would be symptomatic with the foot in plantar flexion, as these fibers could then become impinged within the posterior recess.[23]

Medial STI of the ankle (MSTI), both anterior and posterior in location, is rare and likely involves injury to the deep deltoid ligament. Injury to the deltoid complex only encompasses approximately 15% of all ankle ligamentous pathology.[24] Much of the body of evidence regarding MSTI has only been case reports or case series. Both posteromedial and anteromedial locations have been described; however, the mechanism of injury leading to ligamentous pathology and ankle instability still remains somewhat unclear.[25,26] Koulouris and colleagues[26] found that most injuries leading to posteromedial STI were the inversion type; however, Liu and Mirzayan[27] demonstrated eversion injuries occurring before STI pathology. Although anteromedial STI is more common, both anteromedial and posteromedial STI can exist secondary to tearing of the deep deltoid ligamentous structures, which often leads to laxity in the joint, especially when combined with lateral ligamentous pathology.[26,28] Lateral soft tissue pathology is often present because, as the foot maximally inverts, the talus is in a plantarflexed and internally rotated position. This movement tilts the ankle mortise, which often results in lateral ligament complex tearing or rupture. However, although the MCL complex is strong, Paterson and colleagues[29] suggested that, with a severe inversion injury combined with heavy axial loading of the ankle, the deep posterior fibers of the deltoid ligament could become crushed between the medial malleolus and medial talar allowing to there often being multiple soft tissue pathologies with these types of injuries. Furthermore, many times MSTI is asymptomatic at first, often overshadowed by lateral complex injury or larger pathology associated with ankle pain. Left untreated or insufficiently treated, this allows hypertrophic scar tissue to form and become entrapped within the medial gutter of the ankle leading to impingement with ankle ROM. Additionally, this disorganized mass of tissue can have increased contact forces on the medial articular surface of the talus, which can often lead to changes to the chondromalacia and uneven gliding across the joint surfaces, causing pain.[25,26] Tethering of the flexor tendons secondary to the hypertrophic scar tissue formation can also be associated with MSTI.[26] Although rare, rupture of the deep deltoid ligament without fracture of osseous structures of the ankle has been described in the literature; however, injury to this structure is more commonly associated with multiple pathologies, including malleolar fracture or syndesmotic pathology,[24] often requiring surgical repair. Injuries exhibiting polyaxial loading mechanisms and likely multiple pathologies should be evaluated and treated if present.

CLINICAL PRESENTATION

Historically, patients with ALSTI present with a chief complaint of chronic ankle pain location specific after a single or often multiple inversion or eversion injuries. Many times these patients are athletes who have not been able to resolve their symptoms with standard conservative care. Many times patients will describe a popping or clicking associated with ankle joint ROM and indicate that the pain is increased with prolonged activity. Often times there will be a history of other pathology that was diagnosed at the time of a traumatic event and treated or that was never treated along with the STI.

The physical examination is often benign with regard to ankle instability; however, pinpoint tenderness can be felt on palpation to the respective area of soft tissue pathology, particularly with dorsiflexory ROM. An audible click can sometimes be heard when in a dorsiflexed and everted position, so named the *ankle impingement sign*, and has also been described by Malloy and colleagues[30] for ALSTI with 94.8% and 88.0% sensitivity and specificity, respectively.[30] Generalized swelling and even bruising to the ankle is often present along with a possible palpation of a mass to the anterolateral or anteromedial gutter of the ankle.

Specifically for posteromedial STI, pain on palpation is noted with tenderness identified posterior to the medial malleolus and deep to the posterior tibial tendon.[29] The clinician should be able to differentiate posteromedial STI from anteromedial and osseous pathology by simply placing patients in full passive plantar flexion. This placement will identify boney impingement, such as os trigonum or fracture of the Stieda process, but will be negative with posteromedial or lateral soft tissue pathology.[29]

It should be noted that, although mechanical stability of the ankle is often intact on clinical examination, many patients with STI present with functional instability along with a history of repeated ankle sprains. Some traumatic injuries often have multiple pathologies present, including ligamentous laxity, which leads to ankle instability (mechanical instability) and STI; this can make clinical diagnosis difficult. When ankle instability is also present, multiple procedures may be required to completely treat all symptoms.

DIAGNOSIS

STI syndrome in any location about the ankle must be evaluated in conjunction with a plethora of other possible etiopathologies of ankle pain, including but not limited to osteochondral lesions of the talus, peroneal tendonitis/subluxation, tarsal coalitions, subtalar joint dysfunction, and ligamentous laxity mechanical instability. When found in combination with another pathology, both conservative and surgical treatment options must be all encompassing of the symptoms. A strong history and good clinical examination can often be enough to make the diagnosis. Type of sport or activity can also help lead the clinician to the likely cause. Ultimately, isolated STI often has a somewhat generalized clinical presentation; diagnosis is well aided with the use of ancillary imaging techniques.

IMAGING
Radiographic Analysis

Despite clinical evaluation being most important regarding soft tissue pathology of the ankle, patients are rarely diagnosed without practitioners obtaining some type of advanced diagnostic imaging to aid in their clinical decision-making. Radiographic films are recommended and often ordered with the primary goal to rule out/in osseous pathology. Osseous pathology can be either a primary cause or secondary comorbidity in conjunction with STI, leading to clinical symptoms. Anterior-posterior and lateral radiographs should be taken to evaluate the ankle for tibial or talar spurring as well as to help identify and diagnose possible osteochondral defects (OCDs) in the talocrural joint. Clinical suspicion of posterior pathology is also evaluated with plain radiographs, including ankle impingement secondary to a Haglund-type deformity, a hypertrophic os trigonum, or Stieda process fracture of the posterior aspect of the talus. The superimposition of the medial and lateral posterior processes of the talus, which often occurs with standard radiographic imaging, can sometimes decrease viewing capabilities; it has been suggested that externally rotating the ankle 25° to the normal viewing window may provide a clearer evaluation when pathology is suspected.[31] Furthermore, because of the anteromedial contour of the tibia, osteophytes and OCDs adjacent to the talocrural joint as well as tendon or ligamentous pathology can sometimes be missed or overlooked with plain radiographic imaging; advanced imaging is often indicated. Komenda and Ferkel[32] evaluated 54 patients with chronic ankle instability using arthroscopy and found 93% had intra-articular abnormalities above and beyond STI. Additionally, DiGiovanni and colleagues[4] evaluated 61 patients with chronic ankle instability showing 100% findings of intra-articular abnormalities and 0% findings of isolated lateral ligament injury indicating that patients rarely present with isolated pathology with regard to chronic ankle pain.[4] More commonly, chronic ankle pain, including STI, is likely associated with multiple pathologies suggesting further the need and efficacy of advanced imaging in aiding correct diagnosis in these patient populations.

MRI

MRI is the most useful imaging modality in evaluating as well as excluding soft tissue pathology in the foot and ankle. When using MRI to aid in assessment of ankle impingement, sagittal and coronal T1-weighted, spin echo, short tau inversion recovery or fat-suppressed proton-density images are often the first choice. Axial T2-weighted or proton density–weighted turbo spin-echo sequences are also routinely ordered. MRI is capable of aiding in the diagnosis of fibrosis, thickened synovium, adjacent reactive soft tissue edema, and partial or complete tears of surrounding tendon and ligamentous structures when basic imaging reveals no pathology consistent with the patients' pain.

Despite controversy with some research suggesting that MRI may be less accurate and even ineffective in the diagnosis of ankle STI,[27,33] its efficacy and accuracy for augmenting clinical evaluation of ankle soft tissue pathology has been well documented in the literature. In a study by Lee and colleagues,[34] they found that the use of fat-suppressed contrast enhanced 3-dimensional fat spoiled gradient (CE 3D-FSPGR) had a sensitivity of 91.9%, a specificity of 84.4%, and an accuracy of 87.5% with respect to diagnosing STI.[34] Additionally, Koulouris and colleagues[26] reviewed 25 patients with a history of posteromedial ankle pain comparing multiple advanced imaging studies and concluded that MRI had the ability to access the entire ankle joint.[26] The senior authors think that factors that could affect the ability of MRI to be effective in identifying soft tissue pathology of the ankle includes evaluating anatomy in multiple planes as well as selecting the correct sequence and section thickness of imaging slices based on the location of pathology. They also suggest having no intersection gaps with imaging. Routine MRI slices are 4 mm in size and can be a contributing factor to decreased visibility of soft tissue pathology. Choo and colleagues[35] determined that the use of 3D fat-suppressed MRI with 1.5-mm sectioning was better at lesion characteristic identification than routine magnetic resonance (MR) when looking at anterolateral soft tissue pathology.[35] MR sectioning of 1.5 to 3.0 mm with axial, coronal, and sagittal views is routinely ordered by the senior authors, which they think provides them with excellent viewing capabilities of anteromedial, anterolateral, and posteromedial soft tissue pathology (**Fig. 3**).

Magnetic Resonance Arthrography

The use of MR arthrography (MRA) is also beneficial in the identification of ankle soft tissue pathology; although invasive, it has been identified as the modality for diagnosing ankle impingement.[36,37] Robinson and colleagues[37] found MRA was accurate in assessing anterolateral recess of the ankle with an accuracy of 97%, a sensitivity of 96%, and a specificity of 100%. However, Haller and colleagues evaluated 51 patients with chronic ankle pain comparing MRI versus MRA showing no statistical difference in diagnosing STI of the ankle.[38] This finding, along with the more invasive nature of

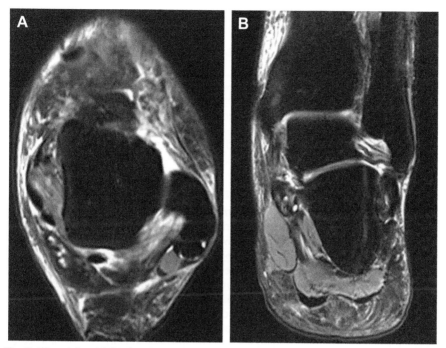

Fig. 3. T2-weighted MRI showing increased signal intensity at the level of the ATFL in the transverse plane indicating likely rupture (*A*). Same pathology shown in the frontal plane (*B*). Transverse plane pathology at the level of the deep deltoid ligament indicating posteromedial STI.

MRA, further supports the senior author's suggestion for using MRI with small sections as the modality of choice for augmenting clinical diagnoses of STI of the ankle.

Ultrasound

The demand for less invasive techniques to aid in diagnosing ankle impingement continues to grow. The evidence in the literature on the efficacy of the use of ultrasound (US) as a viable diagnostic tool is sparse. One study suggested that in comparing MRI with US evaluation, US was as effective in diagnosing posteromedial impingement and may even have an advantage in that it was particularly sensitive in identifying small avulsion fractures that routine MRI may miss.[26] Other studies have described US evaluation in conjunction with US-guided therapeutic injections for STI of the ankle but stated that US was only viable as a single modality after MR has ruled out significant concomitant injuries.[39] Additionally, McCarthy and colleagues[40] evaluated anterolateral STI using US while correlating its findings with clinical assessment and arthroscopic surgical findings. They concluded that it was not only accurate in identifying synovitic lesions within the anterolateral gutter but also in demonstrating findings and differentiation of associated ligamentous and osseous pathology.[40] One other possible advantage to US is its ability to easily evaluate the contralateral limb for comparison of normal fibrillary patterns and correlate results. However, although US may be less invasive and equivalent in comparison with MR with regard to some STI, the inability of US to identify some concomitant ankle pathology, such as OCLs, stress fractures, and even small loose bodies, makes it a difficult unimodality when a differential diagnosis is present clinically.

Radionuclide Imaging and Single-Photon Emission Computed Tomography/Computed Tomography

Other imagining modalities have been described in the literature for aiding the diagnosis of STI in the foot and ankle, including radionuclide and single-photon emission computed tomography/computed tomography imaging. Although these modalities have shown good possibilities for further use, researchers have indicated that they have not been thoroughly evaluated and currently are being used to compliment MR and US imaging techniques.[26,41]

CONSERVATIVE TREATMENT

Often when patients present with symptomology of STI it is usually a chronic course. Many times they have already been treated surgically for other pathology. Initial treatment includes the RINCE pneumonic, which includes rest, ice, antiinflammatory medications, compression, and elevation. Additionally, corticosteroid injections, over-the-counter and custom orthotics, heel lifts, and physical therapy are also introduced as part of the conservative treatment paradigm. Many patients respond well to a combination of physical therapeutic modalities, including proprioceptive training, US or electric stimulation, ROM exercises, and strength training to the surrounding ankle musculature.[42] Patients should be considered surgical candidates when conservative therapy fails over a 3- to 6-month time frame and they continue to have painful symptoms with decreased ROM to the joint surface.[31] However, arthroscopic surgical intervention should also be discussed with patients who may require open procedures at an earlier date because of primary traumatic pathology. In these cases, arthroscopic evaluation and treatment of possible impingement should be completed in conjunction with open procedures to increase the likelihood of good long-term outcomes.

SURGICAL TREATMENT

Ankle arthroscopy is routinely performed in an outpatient setting. The following technique described is often used by the senior author for various anterior soft tissue ankle impingements. The patient is brought into the operating room and placed in a supine position. Following general anesthesia, the patient's limb is often bumped by placing a rolled blanket under the ipsilateral limb. A thigh tourniquet is placed and often times not used when epinephrine is placed in the lactated ringers bag. Both feet are brought to the edge of the table with the heels barely off the table with slight flexion in the knee, as this assists in natural joint distraction. Rarely is a joint distractor used. Following the preparation of the operative extremity using normal sterile aseptic technique, generally above the knee, the medial portal is identified using a spinal needle inserted into the joint. The ankle joint is insufflated with approximately 15 to 18 mL of lactated Ringer solution (LR). The use of an arthroscopy drape is beneficial. Position the viewing monitor to one side of the table for easy visualization for the surgeon. The circulator should then hang a 3-L bag of LR (also including epinephrine) to the intravenous pole for fluid ingress. The egress can be set to gravity or to suction depending on the surgeon's preference.

Following exsanguination and inflation of the thigh tourniquet on the operative extremity, the surgeon should then obtain a marking pen to mark out the arthroscopic portals he or she plans to use. Often 2 portals, the anteromedial and anterolateral portals are sufficient and provide easy access to the more common forms of ankle STI.

Care must be taken when creating the small stab incision with an 11 blade for the anteromedial portal, as the incision should be placed medial to the tibialis anterior tendon and avoid the saphenous nerve and vein. The surgeon should only incise down through the level of the dermis. Blunt dissection should then take place with a straight hemostat to the level of the joint capsule. At this time, a blunt trocar and cannula are inserted and used to penetrate the joint capsule of the ankle joint. The trocar is removed, leaving the cannula in place. Ingress is now started through the cannula using gravity or pressure pump depending on the surgeon's preference. Following this, the camera is introduced through the cannula to gain visualization of the joint space. The authors routinely use a 4.0-mm scope, but a 2.7-mm scope is an alterative sizing option. The anterolateral portal should be done under arthroscopic guidance. Dimming the lights in the operating room can aid in allowing visualization of the lighting mechanism of the camera on the lateral aspect of the ankle and guide location for the lateral stab incision. Before making the lateral incision, the surgeon may insert an 18-gauge needle to confirm anatomic location is superficial to the ankle joint. The 18-gauge needle should be placed lateral to the peroneus tertius tendon, with special care to avoid the neurovascular structures. One should be sure not to make the lateral incision too lateral. Once satisfied with determination of the lateral incision, the needle should be removed and a small stab incision should be performed through the dermal layer. A straight hemostat is then used to dissect to the level of the joint capsule. The capsule is then punctured in similar fashion as with the anteromedial portal placement and the necessary equipment needed to remove the pathology (shaver, electrocautery, burrs and so forth) is inserted with the suction device attached. Debridement of hypertrophied synovium and any thickened fibrous bands are completed using arthroscopic maneuvers including scanning with sweeping, positioning and rotation of the instruments (**Fig. 4**). The equipment can be introduced into either portal depending on location of pathology, allowing better access to debridement. A 4-0 polypropylene (Prolene) suture is then used to reapproximate the skin.

Medial STI lesions are often challenging to access arthroscopically, particularly posteromedial impingement through an anteromedial or anterolateral approach. Many times an arthroscopic procedure is performed anteriorly to assess and treat

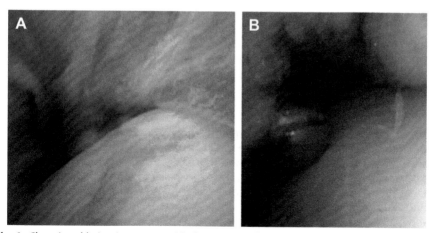

Fig. 4. Chronic ankle impingement with destruction of articular cartilage on the anterior superior lateral talar dome (A); arthroscopic debridement of impinged soft tissue via shaver device (B).

anterior soft tissue pathology; however, posterior arthroscopy is often not attempted for medial lesions because of the inherent safety concerns for surrounding anatomy in the posteromedial portal. Much of the anteromedial and posteromedial lesions are treated with open arthrotomy by the senior authors.

Mosier-La Clair and colleagues'[28] study provides a description of a common surgical approach to anteromedial impingement. The patient is placed in a supine position with the lower extremity in a frog-leg position about the operating table. Once the effected extremity is exsanguinated and the thigh tourniquet is inflated, the deep anterosuperior edge of the deltoid ligament is palpated. Following this, an approximately 3-cm poster-omedial incision is made along its border. Blunt and sharp dissection is carefully completed being sure to protect the surrounding neurovascular structures. Once the ligament is identified, it is isolated and surrounding soft tissue is retracted accordingly. The ligament is then observed while flexing and extending the ankle allowing identification of the STI syndrome. Any hypertrophic synovial tissue and the thickened portion of the ligament is debrided sharply using a scalpel. Occasionally, secondary pathology, such as osteophyte formation, may be visualized and is debrided with a rongeur. The ankle should then be taken through complete ROM to ensure complete removal of STI. The capsule is then reapproximated with absorbable suture material, and the skin is closed in a technique suited to the surgeon's preference.[28]

A similar approach that incorporated an open and arthroscopic technique described by Koulouris and colleagues[26] is also used for posteromedial STI lesions, placing the incision posterior to the medial malleolus and directing it toward the posteromedial fibers of the deep deltoid ligament. In this procedure, the retinaculum is incised over the posterior tibial tendon, soft tissues are retracted, and the deep capsule is identified. Once visualized, the capsule is opened exposing the deep fibers of the deltoid. Hypertrophic-thickened fibers are resected. Koulouris and colleagues[26] then combined this with an arthroscopic approach described by Foetisch and Ferkel[24] using anteromedial, anterolateral, and posterolateral portals to evaluate any further STI pathology.[26] Alternatively, Paterson and colleagues[29] described a technique that gained access to the posteromedial lesion via an incision through the posterior tibial tendon bed. The original incision was made over the posterior tibial tendon approximately 4 cm in length. The lesion was identified through the tendon bed incision and was resected using a scalpel or rongeur. The tendon sheath was repaired, and the skin was closed.[29]

Postoperative course is similar in all procedures and includes non–weight-bearing status often in a posterior splint until sutures are removed. This status is followed by a week of guarded weight bearing with eventual transition back to normal shoe gear as tolerated.

OUTCOMES/COMPLICATIONS

A large body of early clinical data regarding arthroscopic treatment of ALSTI has shown good to excellent results. These results have been well documented in the literature.[42] Ferkel and colleagues[6] reviewed 31 patients retrospectively with a greater than 2-year follow-up showing 85% good to excellent outcomes. Martin and colleagues[43] saw good to excellent outcomes after a 2-year follow-up in 12 to 16 patients. Furthermore, Jacobson and colleagues[42] in 2011 provided a table demonstrating the outcomes of more recent studies, which found good to excellent results ranging from 85% to 91%.

Successful outcomes have also been demonstrated in the adolescent population. As described by Gulish and colleagues,[44] patients who were diagnosed with functional instability of the ankle and underwent arthroscopic intervention were found to have statistically significant changes in American Orthopedic Foot and Ankle Society (AOFAS) scores ranging from 75 to 100 postoperatively. Additionally, Edmonds and colleagues'[45] study of 13 adolescent patients found that nonoperative treatment provided little to no relief of painful symptoms and further found good to excellent results with arthroscopic treatment of ALSTI. Of note, the investigators concluded that, once a diagnosis of ALSTI was made, conservative methods provide little in the way of relief of symptoms and surgical intervention should be considered sooner rather than later in the treatment course.[45]

Medial STI has been less well documented in the literature likely secondary to its rarity. As discussed previously, much of the data comes from individual case reports or case series. Koulouris and colleagues[26] looked at a set of 25 patients who presented with posteromedial ankle pain, with all patients demonstrating scar formation and thickening of the deep deltoid consistent with STI. Twelve of the patients demonstrated tethering of the surrounding tendons and 5 were found to have boney avulsion. Only 12 patients underwent open posterior arthrotomy. In 6 patients, the tendon sheath to the posterior tibial tendon was penetrated, but the tendon was noted to be well preserved. The investigators found that their patients all expressed good relief of pain, with nearly all patients returning to full activity; however, the length of follow-up and time to complete recovery was not noted.[26] Mosier-La Clair and colleagues[28] provided further evidence of good results with surgical treatment of anteromedial impingement. The group evaluated 11 patients with anteromedial STI. All patients underwent open arthrotomy with surgical debridement of the anterior fibers of the deltoid ligament. A large subset of the population had multiple pathologies, including talar dome lesions in 8. With a 4-year follow-up, the investigators reported good to excellent results using the AOFAS scores in 9 patients; it was noted that all patients returned to work. In a series of 6 patients with posteromedial STI presented by Paterson and colleagues,[29] they also found good to excellent results with 100% of patients returning to preinjury level after open arthrotomy and sharp debridement of the hypertrophic-thickened fibers of the deltoid ligament. Arthroscopic debridement of anteromedial STI has also been discussed. Egol and Parisien[25] presented a case report of a patient who presented with chronic pain to the medial ankle and was diagnosed with a partial tear of the deep deltoid ligament. Arthroscopic debridement using the standard anterior portals was completed with excellent results showing no residual detriments at the 1-year follow-up.

Complications arising from arthroscopic only or arthroscopic-assisted surgery with open arthrotomy technique for debridement of STI have been well documented.[42,46–48] Historically, very low complications from ankle arthroscopy have been reported. Zengerink and Van Dijk[47] reported on both anterior and posterior arthroscopic treatment reviewing 1305 patients and found an overall complication rate of 3.5% owing to a dorsiflexion intermittent-distraction technique compared with continuous distraction used by many other series. Recently, Simonson and Roukis[48] completed a systemic review evaluating the overall incidence of complications of arthroscopic treatment of ALSTI. They evaluated 397 ankles with an overall complication rate 4%, indicating that ankle arthroscopy is safe and reliable for treatment of ALSTI (**Table 1**).

Neurologic complications are by far the most common residual deficiency noted after surgery. Ferkel and colleagues[6] demonstrated an overall complication of 10% with differentiation among nerve sheath involvement in their review of 518 patients in 1991. Although Guhl and Schonholtz[49] noted that cutaneous nerve pathology was more common in ankle arthroscopy, there have been multiple descriptions of nerve injury following arthroscopy in other joints in the body as well. Much of the symptoms

Table 1
Overall incidence of complications related to arthroscopic treatment of anterolateral ankle soft tissue impingement, regardless of specific cause, with an overall incidence of complications of 4.0% and an incidence of major complications of 0.8%, indicating that arthroscopy for treating anterior lateral impingement syndrome is a safe and reproducible procedure

Author	Level of Evidence	No. of Patients	No. of Ankles	Mean Age (Range) (y)	Mean Follow-up (Range) (mo)	No. of Major Complications	Total No. of Complications (%)
McCarroll et al, 1987	IV	4	5	NA	24 (12–36)	0	0 (0)
Martin et al, 1989	IV	16	16	28 (12–54)	30 (25–40)	0	3 (18.8)
Bassett et al, 1990	IV	2	2	28 (24–31)	15 (6–24)	0	0 (0)
Ferkel et al, 1991	IV	31	31	34 (16–74)	34 (24–66)	0	0 (0)
Thein & Eichenblat, 1992	IV	3	3	NA	34 (28–44)	0	0 (0)
Meislin et al, 1993	IV	29	29	37 (17–66)	25 (6–41)	0	0 (0)
Liu et al, 1994	IV	55	55	34 (20–67)	31 (12–54)	0	3 (5.5)
Ogilvie-Harris et al, 1997	IV	17	17	29 (17–54)	33 (12–72)	0	0 (0)
DeBerardino et al, 1997	IV	60	60	24 (13–45)	27 (6–64)	0	3 (5)
Akseki et al, 1999	IV	21	21	31 (11–68)	34 (24–48)	2	2 (9.5)
Kim & Ha, 2000	IV	52	52	31 (16–49)	30 (25–45)	0	0 (0)
Urgüden et al, 2005	IV	41	41	33 (15–63)	83.7 (21–152)	1	1 (0.2)
Hassan, 2007	IV	23	23	27 (15–53)	25 (12–38)	0	3 (13)
Koczy et al, 2009	IV	22	22	34 (17–55)	12 (12)	0	1 (4.5)
Moustafa El-Sayed, 2010	IV	20	20	36 (26–49)	21.3 (12–47)	0	0 (0)
Total		396	397	31.2 (11–75)	33.7 (6–152)	3	16 (4)

Abbreviation: NA, not available.
From Simonson DC, Roukis TS. Safety of ankle arthroscopy for the treatment of anterolateral soft-tissue impingement. Arthroscopy 2014;30(2):258; with permission.

associated with nerve injury include hypoesthesia, hyperesthesia, paresthesia, as well as sensory loss or pain at the portal sites. However, these injuries can often be avoided entirely with careful portal placement and anatomic surgical technique.

Infection has also been described in the literature as a complication to arthroscopic surgery. Although the study by Small[50] only showed an infection rate of 0.20% in these types of procedures, the ability for infections to range from the more common superficial nature, to full blown septic arthritis, mandates that extra precautions be taken to minimize the risk of this type of pathology.[46] Aside from sterile technique, correct draping and providing the greatest barrier of sterility possible, attentive postoperative evaluation with early diagnosis and aggressive treatment of possible infection is key to favorable outcomes. Furthermore, although the senior authors use prophylactic antibiotics on a routine basis in ankle arthroscopy, the benefits of their usage remains debated; the evidence-based literature is both dated and sparse.[49,51]

Most complications seen by the senior authors with respect to arthroscopic surgery and arthroscopic-assisted arthrotomy technique have been neuritis in one form or another. The most common causes of neuritis based on the senior author's experience have included poor placement of portals to close to the neurovascular structures, poor fluid balance having more ingress than egress compressing the nerve structures, overzealous debridement of the soft tissues and capsule, and overuse of distraction techniques. Other much less common complications associated with ankle arthroscopy have been thoroughly discussed by Lamy and Stienstra,[46] including but not limited to complex regional pain syndrome, heme-arthrosis, injury to extra-articular structures, thermal injuries, joint effusions, and complications with instrumentation. However, the senior authors think that when performed correctly, taking the steps necessary to guard against adverse outcomes, arthroscopic treatment alone or in combination with open arthrotomy is a safe and reproducible treatment option for STI pathology.

SUMMARY

Chronic STI of the tibiotalar joint often begins with an inciting injury involving a severe inversion–plantar flexion or eversion-dorsiflexion biomechanical pathway. Although inversion and eversion ankle injuries have been reported in both lateral and medial soft tissue pathology, understanding the mechanism of action responsible for primary pathology and completing a strong medical history is paramount to the clinician identifying the correct diagnosis. Loss of either the lateral or medial ligamentous structures responsible for stability of the ankle joint can lead to uncoupling of the foot and tibia ending in gross instability and chronic pain. It has clearly been demonstrated that these types of ankle injuries are often poly-traumatic, and prompt identification and adequate time for healing are required for consistently good long-term results.

Although many people in this patient population do well with conservative treatment, when arthroscopic surgery is indicated as a monotherapy or in conjunction with other procedures, the senior authors think careful preoperative planning and patient selection play a large role in successful treatment. Furthermore, although complications do occur with arthroscopic treatment of STI, the literature has shown very low incidence rates for both anterior and posterior locations, suggesting its safety and reproducibility of good outcomes when performed by trained surgeons.

Ankle sprains or trauma to the ankle joint can lead to injury to the capsule, LCL, LLC, or MCL complex. Identifying inclusion of forced plantar flexion, dorsiflexion, or axial loading as part of the mechanism of injury can help in localizing likely pathology.

Furthermore, rotation of the subtalar joint as a component of the mechanism of injury is likely to be associated more closely with medially based pathology.

STI of the ankle should be suspected in any patients who present with a chief complaint of chronic pain secondary to an injury or sprain. Most commonly, impinged structures secondary to injury to the ligamentous constructs of the ankle induce formation of scar and inflammatory tissue. When conservative treatment options fail, arthroscopy as a monotherapy and sometimes combined with open resection of this pathology is an effective treatment paradigm that has produced good to excellent long-term results.

REFERENCES

1. Billi A, Catalucci A, Barile A, et al. Joint impingement syndrome: clinical features. Eur J Radiol 1998;27(Suppl 1):S39–41.
2. Morris LH. Report of cases of athlete's ankle. J Bone Joint Surg 1943;25:220.
3. Balduni FC, Tetzlaff J. Historical perspectives on injuries of the ligaments of the ankle. Clin Sports Med 1982;1(1):3–12.
4. DiGiovanni BF, Fraga CJ, Cohen BE, et al. Associated injuries found in chronic lateral ankle instability. Foot Ankle Int 2000;21(10):809–15.
5. Smith RW, Reischl SF. Treatment of ankle sprains in young athletes. Am J Sports Med 1986;14(6):465–71.
6. Ferkel RD, Karzel RP, Del Pizzo W, et al. Arthroscopic treatment of anterolateral impingement of the ankle. Am J Sports Med 1991;19(5):440–6.
7. Van Dijk CN. Ankle impingement. In: Chan KM, Karlsson J, editors. ISAKOS/FIMS World consensus conference on ankle instability. Stockholm (Sweden): SAGE; 2005. p. 68–9.
8. Wolin I, Glassman F, Sideman S. Internal derangement of the talofibular component of the ankle. Surg Gynecol Obstet 1950;91:193–200.
9. Urguden M, Soyuncu Y, Ozemir H, et al. Arthroscopic treatment of anterolateral soft tissue impingement of the ankle: evaluation of factors affecting outcome. Arthroscopy 2005;21:317–22.
10. Amendola A, Petrik J, Webster-Bogaert S. Ankle arthroscopy: outcome in 79 consecutive patients. Arthroscopy 1996;12(5):565–73.
11. Lundeen RO. Ankle arthroscopy in the adolescent patient. J Foot Surg 1990; 29(5):510–5.
12. Nikolopoulos CE. Anterolateral instability of the ankle joint. An anatomical, experimental and clinical study (dissertation). Athens (Greece): University of Athens; 1982.
13. Bassett FH 3rd, Gates HS 3rd, Billys JB, et al. Talar impingement by the anteroinferior tibiofibular ligament. A cause of chronic pain in the ankle after inversion sprain. J Bone Joint Surg Am 1990;72(1):55–9.
14. Ray RG, Kriz BM. Anterior inferior tibiofibular ligament. Variations and relationship to the talus. J Am Podiatr Med Assoc 1991;81:479–85.
15. Akseki D, Pinar H, Yaldiz K, et al. The anterior tibiofibular ligament and talar impingement: a cadaveric study. Knee Surg Sports Traumatol Arthrosc 2002; 10:321–6.
16. van den Bekerom MPJ, Raven EEJ. The distal fascicle of the anterior inferior tibiofibular ligament as a cause of tibiotalar impingement syndrome: a current concepts review. Knee Surg Sports Traumatol Arthrosc 2007;15(4):465–71.
17. Johnson EE, Markolf KL. The contribution of the anterior talofibular ligament to ankle laxity. J Bone Joint Surg Am 1983;65(1):81–8.

18. Nikolopoulos CE, Tsirikos AI, Sourmelis S, et al. The accessory anteroinferior ti-biofibular ligament as a cause of talar impingement: a cadaveric study. Am J Sports Med 2004;32(2):389–95.

19. Golanó P, Mariani PP, Rodriguez-Neidenfuhr M, et al. Arthroscopic anatomy of the posterior ankle ligaments. Arthroscopy 2002;18(4):353–8.

20. Golanó P, Vega J, Pérez-Carro L, et al. Ankle anatomy for the arthroscopist. Part II: role of the ankle ligaments in soft tissue impingement. Foot Ankle Clin 2006; 11(2):275–96, v–vi.

21. Chen Y. Arthroscopy of the ankle joint. In: Watanabe M, editor. Arthroscopy of small joints. New York: Igaku-Shoin; 1985. p. 104–27.

22. Hamilton WG, Geppert MJ, Thompson FM. Pain in the posterior aspect of the ankle in dancers. Differential diagnosis and operative treatment. J Bone Joint Surg 1996;78(10):1491–500.

23. Peace KAL, Hillier JC, Hulme A, et al. MRI features of posterior ankle impinge-ment syndrome in ballet dancers: a review of 25 cases. Clin Radiol 2004;59: 1025–33.

24. Foetisch CA, Ferkel RD. Deltoid ligament injuries; anatomy diagnosis and treat-ment. Sports Med Arthrosc Rev 2000;8:326–35.

25. Egol KA, Parisien JS. Impingement syndrome of the ankle caused by a medial meniscoid lesion. Arthroscopy 1997;13(4):522–5.

26. Koulouris G, Connell D, Schneider T, et al. Posterior tibiotalar injury resulting in posteromedial impingement. Foot Ankle Int 2003;24(8):575–83.

27. Liu SH, Mirzayan R. Posteromedial ankle impingement. Arthroscopy 1993;9(6): 709–11.

28. Mosier-La Clair SM, Monroe MT, Manoli A. Medial impingement syndrome of the anterior tibiotalar fascicle of the deltoid ligament on the talus. Foot Ankle Int 2000; 21(5):385–91.

29. Paterson RS, Brown JN, Roberts SMJ. The posteromedial impingement lesion of the ankle. A series of six cases. Am J Sports Med 2001;29(5):550–7.

30. Molloy S, Solan MC, Bendall SP. Synovial impingement in the ankle. A new phys-ical sign. J Bone Joint Surg Br 2003;85(3):330–3.

31. Tol JL, Niek van Dijk C. Anterior ankle impingement. Foot Ankle Clin 2006;11(2): 297–310.

32. Komenda GA, Ferkel RD. Arthroscopic findings associated with the unstable ankle. Foot Ankle Int 1999;20(11):708–13.

33. Farookie S, Yao L, Seeger LL. Anterolateral impingement of the ankle: effective-ness of MR imaging. Radiology 1998;207(2):357–60.

34. Lee JW, Suh JS, Huh YM, et al. Soft tissue impingement syndrome of the ankle: diagnostic efficacy of MRI and clinical results after arthroscopic treatment. Foot Ankle Int 2004;25(12):896–902.

35. Choo HJ, Suh JS, Kim SJ, et al. Ankle MRI for anterolateral soft tissue impinge-ment: increased accuracy with the use of contrast-enhanced fat-suppressed 3D-FSPGR MRI. Korean J Radiol 2008;9(5):409–15.

36. Robinson P, White LM, Salonen D, et al. Anteromedial impingement of the ankle: using MR arthrography to assess the anteromedial recess. Am J Roentgenol 2002;178(3):601–4.

37. Robinson P, White LM, Salonen DC, et al. Anterolateral ankle Impingement: MR arthrographic assessment of the anterolateral recess 1. Radiology 2001;221: 1186–90.

38. Haller J, Bernt R, Seeger T, et al. MR-imaging of anterior tibiotalar impingement syndrome: agreement, sensitivity and specificity of MR-imaging and indirect MR-arthrography. Eur J Radiol 2006;58(3):450–60.

39. Messiou C, Robinson P, O'Connor PJ, et al. Subacute posteromedial impingement of the ankle in athletes: MR imaging evaluation and ultrasound guided therapy. Skeletal Radiol 2006;35(2):88–94.

40. McCarthy CL, Wilson DJ, Coltman TP. Anterolateral ankle impingement: findings and diagnostic accuracy with ultrasound imaging. Skeletal Radiol 2008;37(3):209–16.

41. Chicklore S, Gnanasegaran G, Vijayanathan S, et al. Potential role of multislice SPECT/CT in impingement syndrome and soft-tissue pathology of the ankle and foot. Nucl Med Commun 2013;34(2):130–9.

42. Jacobson K, Ng A, Haffner KE. Arthroscopic treatment of anterior ankle impingement. Clin Podiatr Med Surg 2011;28(3):491–510.

43. Martin DF, Baker CL, Curl WW, et al. Operative ankle arthroscopy Long-term follow-up. Am J Sports Med 1989;17(1):16–23.

44. Gulish HA, Sullivan RJ, Aronow M. Arthroscopic treatment of soft-tissue impingement lesions of the ankle in adolescents. Foot Ankle Int 2005;26(3):204–7.

45. Edmonds EW, Chambers R, Kaufman E, et al. Anterolateral ankle impingement in adolescents: outcomes of nonoperative and operative treatment. J Pediatr Orthop 2010;30(2):186–91.

46. Lamy C, Stienstra JJ. Complications in ankle arthroscopy. Clin Podiatr Med Surg 1994;11(3):523–39.

47. Zengerink M, van Dijk CN. Complications in ankle arthroscopy. Knee Surg Sports Traumatol Arthrosc 2012;20(8):1420–31.

48. Simonson DC, Roukis TS. Safety of ankle arthroscopy for the treatment of anterolateral soft-tissue impingement. Arthroscopy 2014;30(2):256–9.

49. Guhl JF, Schonholtz GJ. Complications and prevention. In: Guhl JF, editor. Foot and ankle arthroscopy. 2nd edition. Thorofare (NJ): SpringerLink; 1993. p. 215.

50. Small NC. Complications in arthroscopic surgery performed by experienced arthroscopists. Arthroscopy 1988;4(3):215–21.

51. D'Angelo GL, Ogilvie-Harris DJ. Septic arthritis following arthroscopy, with cost/benefit analysis of antibiotic prophylaxis. Arthroscopy 1988;4(1):10–4.

Arthroscopic Management of Osteochondral Lesions of the Talus

Sean T. Grambart, DPM

KEYWORDS

- Osteochondral lesions • Talar dome lesion • Microfracture • Articular damage
- Ankle impingement

KEY POINTS

- Size of the osteochondral lesion seems to be the indicator of success. Small osteochondral lesions fair best with microfracture techniques.
- Microfracture technique involves perforating the subchondral plate 3 to 4 mm in depth and spaced 3 to 4 mm apart.
- Controversy exist with postoperative management of osteochondral lesions.

It is estimated that 1 in 10,000 people sustain an ankle injury every day, with the incidence as high a 9.35 in 10,000 in athletes during active competition.[1] Osteochondral fractures of the ankle are typically caused by traumatic injuries. Traumatic injuries have been reported to be associated with 70% of medial and 98% of lateral osteochondral lesions of the talus.[2] It has been reported that up to 50% of ankle sprains and 73% of ankle fractures can have associated osteochondral injuries.[3–5] Given that cartilage has a poor tendency to heal because it is avascular, as the population continues to be more active, it can be assumed that osteochondral lesions will become more prevalent. Repetitive trauma can lead to further cartilage damage, with subsequent increasing size of the lesion ultimately leading to severe cartilage disorder and degenerative arthritis of the ankle.[6,7]

In the acute setting with ankle injuries, osteochondral defect can often be overlooked because of similar symptoms of ankle sprains, such as ankle pain, swelling, and limited range of motion. Most typical ankle sprain symptoms resolve after about 4 to 6 weeks. With lingering symptoms, osteochondral injuries should be suspected. Chronic pain along the ankle joint, especially on the medial and lateral gutters, can be associated with osteochondral injuries. Clinical findings such as locking or clicking in the joint are typical but are not absolute in the presentation of osteochondral lesions.[8,9]

Carle Physician Group, Department of Orthopedics, 1802 South Mattis Avenue, Champaign, IL 61821, USA
E-mail address: Sean.Grambart@Carle.com

Clin Podiatr Med Surg 33 (2016) 521–530
http://dx.doi.org/10.1016/j.cpm.2016.06.008
0891-8422/16/$ – see front matter © 2016 Elsevier Inc. All rights reserved.

The treatment of osteochondral lesions depends on the characteristics of the lesions, such as the location, the depth, bone involvement, arthroscopic access, and cartilage involvement. Locations of osteochondral lesions have been studied extensively and both medial and lateral lesions are common. In their classic article, Berndt and Harty[10] reported that the most common locations for osteochondral lesions were posterior-medial at 57% and anterior-lateral at 43%.

More recently, the locations of the common lesions described by Berndt and Harty[10] have been challenged. Elias and colleagues[11] performed a study to evaluate the incidence of osteochondral lesions on the talar dome by location and by morphologic characteristics on MRI (**Fig. 1**). They established a novel, 9-zone anatomic grid system on the talar dome for an accurate depiction of lesion location. The 9 zones on the talar dome articular surface have an equal 3 × 3 grid configuration. Zone 1 was the most anterior and medial, zone 3 was anterior and lateral, zone 7 was most posterior and medial, and zone 9 was the most posterior and lateral. The grid was designed with all 9 zones being equal in surface area. Two observers reviewed MRI examinations of 428 ankles in 424 patients with reported osteochondral talar lesions. Frequency of involvement and size of lesion for each zone were recorded. The medial talar dome was more frequently involved at 62% compared with the lateral talar dome at 34%. In the anterior to posterior direction, the center of the talus was much more frequently involved at 80% than the anterior (6%) and posterior (14%). Center-medial was most common at 53% followed by center-lateral at 26%. Lesions in the medial third of the talar dome were significantly larger in surface area involvement and deeper than those at the lateral talar dome.

One of the most important factors is the quality of the bone and prognostic factors. Nakasa and colleagues[12] evaluated the relationship between arthroscopic findings

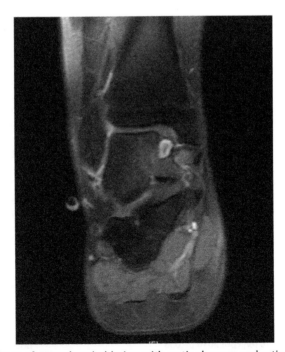

Fig. 1. MRI findings of osteochondral lesion with cystic changes and articular damage.

and computed tomography (CT) scans of osteochondral lesions. Patients underwent CT, MRI, and arthroscopic surgery. The 3 types for the cystic lesion ankles were irregular shape, round shape with sclerotic wall, and irregular shape with opening to an articular cavity. The 3 types for the fragment lesions were no bone absorption, bed absorption without fragment absorption, and bed sclerosis and fragment absorption. Results showed that all round and sclerotic cystic lesions revealed cartilaginous flap lesions with a nearly normal cartilage surface. An irregular shape with opening revealed an unstable lesion with severely damaged cartilage. For fragment lesions, no absorption revealed a stable lesion with a nearly normal cartilage surface. Bed absorption revealed an unstable lesion with a nearly normal cartilage surface. Fragment absorption with bed sclerosis showed an unstable lesion with severely damaged cartilage. The investigators concluded that the diagnosis of cartilage status by CT was better than MRI (**Fig. 2**).

The size of the lesion plays a significant role in the success of surgical intervention. Large lesions with cystic changes have a decreased success rate. Choi and colleagues[13] evaluated factors associated with favorable or unfavorable outcomes with marrow stimulation. The hypothesis is that a defect size may exist at which clinical outcomes become poor in the treatment of osteochondral lesion of the talus. One-hundred and twenty ankles underwent arthroscopic marrow stimulation treatment of osteochondral lesions of the talus and were evaluated for prognostic factors. Clinical

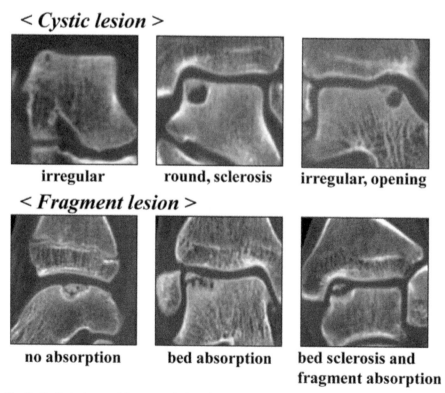

< Cystic lesion >

| irregular | round, sclerosis | irregular, opening |

< Fragment lesion >

| no absorption | bed absorption | bed sclerosis and fragment absorption |

Fig. 2. Cystic lesion and fragment lesion. (*From* Nakasa T, Adachi N, Kato T, et al. Appearance of subchondral bone in computed tomography is related to cartilage damage in osteochondral lesions of the talar dome. Foot Ankle Int 2014;35(6):604; with permission.)

failure was defined as patients having osteochondral transplantation or an American Orthopedic Foot and Ankle Society (AOFAS) Ankle-Hindfoot Scale score less than 80. The investigators used linear regression analysis and the Kaplan-Meier method was used to identify optimal cutoff values of defect size. Eight ankles (6.7%) required osteochondral transplantation, and 22 ankles (18.4%) were considered failures because of AOFAS scores less than 80, which indicated fair or poor results. Linear regression analysis showed a high prognostic significance of defect area and suggested a cutoff defect size of 150 mm^2 for the optimum identification of poor clinical outcomes ($P<.001$). Only 10 of 95 ankles (10.5%) with a defect area less than 150 mm^2 showed clinical failure, whereas in patients with an area greater than or equal to 150 mm^2 the clinical failure rate was significantly higher (80%, 20 of 25). There was no association between outcome and the patient's age, duration of symptoms, trauma, associated lesions, and location of lesions ($P>.05$). The investigators concluded that initial defect size is an important and easily obtainable prognostic factor in osteochondral lesions of the talus and so may serve as a basis for preoperative surgical decisions. A cutoff point exists regarding the risk of clinical failure at a defect area of approximately 150 mm^2 (**Fig. 3**).[13]

Yoshimura and colleagues[14] studied the prognostic factors for small osteochondral lesions of the talus with a bone marrow stimulation technique. They evaluated 50 ankles in 50 patients treated with arthroscopic bone marrow stimulation techniques for an osteochondral lesion of the talus (<150 mm^2). The mean lesion size was 62 mm^2 (range, 7–119 mm^2). The mean AOFAS score improved from 74 (range, 18–90) preoperatively to 90 (range, 67–100) postoperatively. Linear regression analyses showed prognostic significance for lesion depth and outcome. Medial lesions had a significantly higher incidence of poor outcomes than lateral lesions ($P<.05$). Among the medial lesions, lesions uncovered with the medial malleolus had inferior outcomes

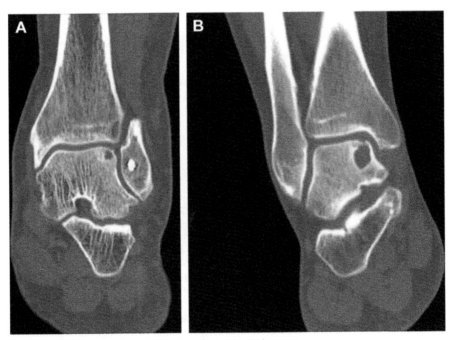

Fig. 3. Small (*A*) versus large (*B*) lesion shown in CT images.

compared with covered lesions ($P<.0001$). There was no association between clinical outcome and lesion size or body mass index. In older patients ($\geq$40 years), there was a significant trend toward inferior clinical outcomes ($P<.05$). The investigators concluded that arthroscopic bone marrow stimulation techniques provided satisfactory clinical outcomes. However, older patients, deep lesions, and medial lesions uncovered with the medial malleolus were associated with inferior clinical outcomes.

Chuckpaiwong and colleagues[15] reported a 100% success rate in patients with lesions smaller than 15 mm in diameter. One-hundred and five consecutive patients with osteochondral lesions of the ankle who underwent ankle arthroscopy with microfracture were prospectively followed up for a mean of 31.6 ± 12.1 months. Subjects were evaluated at 6 weeks, 3 months, 6 months, 12 months, and annually after surgery. There were no failures of treatment with lesions smaller than 15 mm. In contrast, only 1 patient met the criteria for success in the group of lesions greater than 15 mm. Besides size, other factors, including increasing age, higher body mass index, history of trauma, and presence of osteophytes, negatively affected outcome. The presence of instability and the presence of anterolateral soft tissue scar were correlated with a successful outcome. The investigators found a strong correlation between lesion size and success across the population. For lesions smaller than 15 mm, regardless of location, excellent results were obtained.

ARTHROSCOPIC TREATMENT

The goal of surgical management of an osteochondral fracture is to create a stable cartilage environment, eliminate pain, and restore the function of the ankle. Techniques for surgical management of osteochondral lesions consist of bone marrow stimulation, autologous chondrocyte implantation, matrix autologous chondrocyte implantation, and particulated juvenile cartilage allograft.

Bone marrow stimulation is often used as the first line of treatment. The procedure has the advantages of cost-effectiveness, simplicity of procedure, low complication rate, and low postoperative pain compared with more invasive open procedures. The primary indication for arthroscopic bone marrow stimulation repair is for small, noncystic lesions. Marrow stimulation techniques involve microfracture or drilling of the subchondral plate. Penetrating the subchondral plates allows mesenchymal cells and growth factors to migrate to the area. Growth factors and an initial fibrin clot form to create fibrocartilage, primarily over the first 6 weeks. Fibrocartilage from microfracture, composed primarily of type 1 collagen, has inferior biological and biomechanical properties compared with normal hyaline cartilage.[16,17]

The author's preferred surgical technique is an outpatient procedure. General anesthetic is commonly used with a thigh tourniquet. Three blankets are placed under the operative leg, although leg holders are commonly used as well. The foot should be hanging off the edge of the blanket or leg holders. The external ankle anatomy is marked, including the tip of the medial malleolus, medial aspect of the tibialis anterior tendon, and the superficial peroneal nerve. The anterior-medial incision is marked. The joint is insufflated with lactated Ringer. This insufflation also allows good portal placement to be ensured.

Anterior-lateral and anterior-medial portals are established given access to the joint. Once all of the soft tissue disorder has been debrided, the articular surface can be evaluated. Probes are used to identify the cartilage defects. Most of the osteochondral lesions have defects in the cartilage. Any loose or lifting pieces of cartilage need to be resected via a curette or shaver (**Fig. 4**). In some lesions, the overlying cartilage is

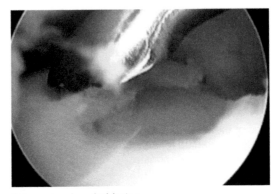

Fig. 4. Curettage of the osteochondral lesion.

intact but has a soft spot or a trampoline appearance. In cases of this trampoline lesion (**Fig. 5**), I use a retrograde approach to try to preserve the intact hyaline cartilage.

With the loose pieces of cartilage removed, the defect is exposed. Gently take a curette and scrape the subchondral plate to remove any loose fragments and to prepare the bed. Microfracture or drilling the defect is performed by perforating the subchondral plate. The perforations created in the subchondral bone allow the blood to form a fibrin clot and release cytokines and growth factors.[18,19]

The marrow stimulation technique is done by placing instrument at 90° to the subchondral plate (**Fig. 6**). The perforations should be placed 3 to 4 mm apart. Once the subchondral plate is adequately perforated, take the shaver and position it over the defect to remove any loose pieces of bone or cartilage to prevent loose bodies within the ankle (**Fig. 7**). Stop the fluid and check for adequate bleeding from the perforations (**Fig. 8**). If there is no bleeding from the perforations, I often switch to a Kirschner wire to increase the depth of the bone penetration. Some studies advocate marrow stimulation in combination with the use of bone marrow aspirate and platelet-rich plasma

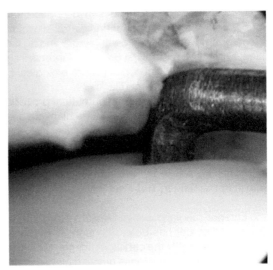

Fig. 5. Soft but intact cartilage giving the trampoline effect.

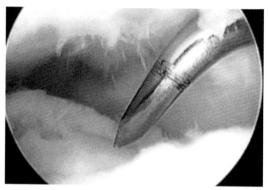

Fig. 6. Perforation of the osteochondral lesion.

to improve the environment for cartilage healing.[20] Even synovial fluid in the ankle joint can be a source of mesenchymal cells. Synovial fluid collected from the ankle joints has shown that human synovial fluid is a good source of mesenchymal stem cells, with the capacity to differentiate into several cell lineages.[21]

There is debate on the length of time for non–weight bearing after a marrow stimulation procedure. The traditional protocol is 6 weeks non–weight bearing. However, studies have challenged this thinking. Dong-Hyun Lee and colleagues[22] performed a prospective, randomized study to compare the clinical results of early and delayed weight bearing after microfracture of small to midsized osteochondral lesions of the talus. Eighty-one ankles in 81 patients with a single osteochondral lesion of the talus that had been treated by arthroscopic microfracture constituted the study cohort. Ankles were allocated to either a delayed weight bearing (DWB) group (41 ankles) or an early weight bearing (EWB) group (40 ankles). Postoperatively, patients in the DWB group maintained non–weight bearing for 6 weeks, but the EWB group was allowed early weight bearing (as tolerated) at 2 weeks. Mean AOFAS ankle-hindfoot scores were 64.9 points in the DWB group and 66.5 points in the EWB group preoperatively, and these improved to 89.5 and 89.3 at the final follow-up visits, respectively. The study shows that early weight bearing postoperative regimens can be recommended

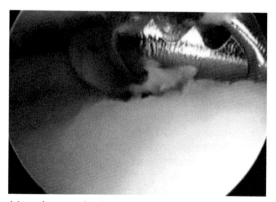

Fig. 7. Shaver positioned over the lesion to remove any loose cartilage or osseous fragments.

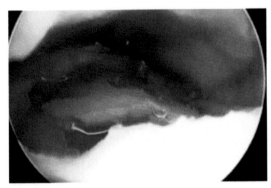

Fig. 8. Adequate vascular inflow from the perforations.

for patients treated by microfracture for small to midsized osteochondral lesions of the talus.

The author's preferred postoperative course is typically 2 weeks non–weight bearing, followed by 4 weeks in a walking boot. At that point, patients start to transition out of the boot and into a shoe, but I still recommend low-impact activities until about 4 months postoperatively, and then patients can start to advance activities as tolerated.

RESULTS

Recent studies have shown that arthroscopic bone marrow stimulation can yield good results. Polat and colleagues[23] assessed the long-term clinical and radiographic outcomes of arthroscopic debridement and microfracture for osteochondral lesions of the talus. Eighty-two patients who were treated with arthroscopic debridement and microfracture for osteochondral lesions of the talus between 1996 and 2009 with a minimum 5-year follow-up were included in the study group. Functional scores (AOFAS, VAS [Visual Analogue Score]) and ankle range of motion were determined, and an arthrosis evaluation was performed. Subgroup evaluations based on age, lesion localization, and defect size were performed using functional outcome correlations. The mean preoperative AOFAS score was 58.7 ± 5.2 (49–75), and the mean postoperative AOFAS score was 85.5 ± 9.9 (56–100). At the last follow-up, 35 patients (42.6%) had no symptoms and 19 patients (23.1%) had pain after walking for more than 2 hours or after competitive sports activities. Radiological assessments of arthrosis revealed that no patient had grade 4 arthritis but that 27 patients (32.9%) had a 1-stage increase in their arthrosis level. Subgroup analyses of the lesion location showed that lateral lesions had significantly better functional results ($P = .02$). The investigators concluded that arthroscopic debridement and microfracture provide a good option for the treatment of osteochondral lesions of the talus over the long term in select patients. Functional outcomes did not correlate with defect size or patient age. Orthopedic surgeons should adopt the microfracture technique, which is minimally invasive and effective for treating osteochondral lesions of the talus.

Hannon and colleagues[24] compared retrospective functional and MRI outcomes after arthroscopic bone marrow stimulation with and without concentrated bone marrow aspirate as a biological adjunct to the surgical treatment of osteochondral lesions of the talus. They found that bone marrow stimulation is an effective treatment strategy for treatment of osteochondral lesions of the talus and results in good medium-term functional outcomes. Arthroscopic bone marrow stimulation with bone marrow aspirate also results in similar functional outcomes and improved border repair tissue integration, with less evidence of fissuring and fibrillation on MRI.

SUMMARY

Arthroscopic bone marrow stimulation has been shown to be a highly successful option for patients with small osteochondral lesions. Studies show a higher failure rate for larger lesions and cystic changes that disrupt the subchondral plate. The threshold size seems to be 150 mm^2.

REFERENCES

1. Nelson AJ, Collins CL, Yard EE, et al. Ankle injuries among United States high school sports athletes, 2005-2006. J Athl Train 2007;42(3):381–7.
2. Loren GJ, Ferkel RD. Arthroscopic assessment of occult intra-articular injury in acute ankle fractures. Arthroscopy 2002;18(4):412–21.
3. Savage-Elliott I, Ross KA, Smyth NA, et al. Osteochondral lesions of the talus: a current concepts review and evidence-based treatment paradigm. Foot Ankle Spec 2014;7(5):414–22.
4. Saxena A, Eakin C. Articular talar injuries in athletes: results of microfracture and autogenous bone graft. Am J Sports Med 2007;35(10):1680–7.
5. Soboroff SH, Pappius EM, Komaroff AL. Benefits, risks, and costs of alternative approaches to the evaluation and treatment of severe ankle sprain. Clin Orthop Relat Res 1984;(183):160–8.
6. Jackson DW, Lalor PA, Aberman HM, et al. Spontaneous repair of full-thickness defects of articular cartilage in a goat model. A preliminary study. J Bone Joint Surg Am 2001;83-A(1):53–64.
7. Mankin HJ. The response of articular cartilage to mechanical injury. J Bone Joint Surg Am 1982;64(3):460–6.
8. McCollum GA, Calder JD, Longo UG, et al. Talus osteochondral bruises and defects: diagnosis and differentiation. Foot Ankle Clin 2013;18(1):35–47.
9. Zengerink M, Szerb I, Hangody L, et al. Current concepts: treatment of osteochondral ankle defects. Foot Ankle Clin 2006;11(2):331–59, vi.
10. Berndt AL, Harty M. Transchondral fractures (osteochondritis dissecans) of the talus. J Bone Joint Surg Am 1959;41-A:988–1020.
11. Elias I, Zoga AC, Morrison WB, et al. Osteochondral lesions of the talus: localization and morphologic data from 424 patients using a novel anatomical grid scheme. Foot Ankle Int 2007;28(2):154–61.
12. Nakasa T, Adachi N, Kato T, et al. Appearance of subchondral bone in computed tomography is related to cartilage damage in osteochondral lesions of the talar dome. Foot Ankle Int 2014;35(6):600–6.
13. Choi WJ, Park KK, Kim BS, et al. Osteochondral lesion of the talus: is there a critical defect size for poor outcome? Am J Sports Med 2009;37(10):1974–80.
14. Yoshimura I, Kanazawa K, Takeyama A, et al. Arthroscopic bone marrow stimulation techniques for osteochondral lesions of the talus: prognostic factors for small lesions. Am J Sports Med 2013;41(3):528–34.
15. Chuckpaiwong B, Berkson EM, Theodore GH. Microfracture for osteochondral lesions of the ankle: outcome analysis and outcome predictors of 105 cases. Arthroscopy 2008;24(1):106–12.

16. Murawski CD, Foo LF, Kennedy JG. A review of arthroscopic bone marrow stimulation techniques of the talus: the good, the bad, and the causes for concern. Cartilage 2010;1(2):137–44.
17. Nehrer S, Spector M, Minas T. Histologic analysis of tissue after failed cartilage repair procedures. Clin Orthop Relat Res 1999;(365):149–62.
18. Buckwalter JA, Mow VC, Ratcliffe A. Restoration of injured or degenerated articular cartilage. J Am Acad Orthop Surg 1994;2(4):192–201.
19. DePalma AF, McKeever CD, Subin DK. Process of repair of articular cartilage demonstrated by histology and autoradiography with tritiated thymidine. Clin Orthop Relat Res 1966;48:229–42.
20. Kennedy JG, Murawski CD. The treatment of osteochondral lesions of the talus with autologous osteochondral transplantation and bone marrow aspirate concentrate: surgical technique. Cartilage 2011;2(4):327–36.
21. Kim YS, Lee HJ, Yeo JE, et al. Isolation and characterization of human mesenchymal stem cells derived from synovial fluid in patients with osteochondral lesion of the talus. Am J Sports Med 2015;43(2):399–406.
22. Lee DH, Lee KB, Jung ST, et al. Erratum. Am J Sports Med 2012;40(10):NP28.
23. Polat G, Erşen A, Erdil ME, et al. Long-term results of microfracture in the treatment of talus osteochondral lesions. Knee Surg Sports Traumatol Arthrosc 2016;24(4):1299–303.
24. Hannon CP, Ross KA, Murawski CD, et al. Arthroscopic bone marrow stimulation and concentrated bone marrow aspirate for osteochondral lesions of the talus: a case-control study of functional and magnetic resonance observation of cartilage repair tissue outcomes. Arthroscopy 2016;32(2):339–47.

Arthroscopic Approach to Posterior Ankle Impingement

Michael H. Theodoulou, DPM*, Laura Bohman, DPM

KEYWORDS

- Posterior ankle impingement • Arthroscopic • Endoscopic • Os trigonum

KEY POINTS

- Posterior ankle pain can occur for many reasons. If it is produced by forced plantarflexion of the foot, it is often a result of impingement from an enlarged posterior talar process or the presence of an accessory ossicle, known as an os trigonum. This condition may present in either the acute or chronic state.
- Management is initially nonoperative but, if pain remains refractory, then surgical treatments are available. Because this is a condition often seen in athletes, procedures that limit surgical trauma and allow early return to activity are ideal.
- Arthroscopic approach for this disorder has been shown to produce good to excellent outcomes with limited complications. Understanding the indications, local anatomy, and surgical technique allows good reproducible outcomes.

 Video content accompanies this article at http://www.podiatric.theclinics.com.

INTRODUCTION

Posterior impingement syndrome is often synonymous with the terms posterior talar compression syndrome, os trigonum syndrome, posterior ankle block, nutcracker-type impingement, and posterior tibiotalar impingement syndrome. Frequently, it is associated with the presence of an accessory ossicle known as the os trigonum. Pain can be elicited acutely with a forced plantarflexion injury or chronically in those individuals performing repetitive plantarflexory moments of the foot and ankle, such as ballerinas or soccer players. The latter presentation is more common.

The os trigonum develops as a secondary cartilaginous center during the second month of fetal development, between the ages of 7 and 11 years in girls and 11 and 13 years in boys. Through enchondral ossification, the center fuses to the postero-lateral talus with a cartilaginous synchondrosis.[1] One year after its appearance, the

Department of Surgery, Cambridge Health Alliance, 1493 Cambridge Street, Cambridge, MA 02139, USA
* Corresponding author.
E-mail address: mtheodoulou@challiance.org

Clin Podiatr Med Surg 33 (2016) 531–543
http://dx.doi.org/10.1016/j.cpm.2016.06.009   **podiatric.theclinics.com**
0891-8422/16/$ – see front matter © 2016 Elsevier Inc. All rights reserved.

secondary center unites to the talar body producing the Stieda process.[2] Failure to unite has been identified in 1.7% to 49%[3] of the general population. Intimate to the presence of this accessory ossicle, is the flexor hallucis longus (FHL) tendon. As a result, the tendon is susceptible to a stenosis tenosynovitis. Chronic entrapment of this tendon can occur resulting from low-lying muscle tissue, impingement from an os trigonum, and incongruity of maximum plantarflexion and dorsiflexion of the ankle and great toe joint resulting in compression of the tendon. This condition often occurs in the fibro-osseous tunnel posterior to the medial malleolus. This condition can be seen in athletes who require forceful plantarflexion of the foot, such as soccer players, swimmers, and ice skaters.

ANATOMY

The posterior ankle joint complex is well defined by soft tissue and osseous structures. Medially, it is bounded by the flexor tendons of the leg, including (from superficial to deep) the posterior tibial tendon, the flexor digitorum longus, and the FHL. The FHL tendon is a critical medial boundary during arthroscopy because the neurovascular bundle lies just medial or posterior to this structure (**Fig. 1**). Posteriorly, the prominent Achilles tendon is appreciated. Laterally, the peroneal tendons serve as an outside boundary to protect the sural nerve and small saphenous vein during arthroscopy. Anteriorly lies the tibiotalar and talocalcaneal joints. Inferiorly, is the tuber of the calcaneus. Within the contents of this vault is adipose tissue frequently refer to as the Kager triangle.

In 2002, Sitler and colleagues[4] published an anatomic study regarding structures at risk when performing posterior ankle arthroscopy through both medial and lateral portals. They examined 13 fresh frozen cadavers and placed plastic cannulas filled with oil in portals to serve as landmarks when performing MRI. Imaging studies were compared with open dissection of the specimens to confirm correlation of proximity of vital structures. Portals were placed immediately adjacent to the Achilles tendon. It was appreciated that, on average, the sural nerve was 3.2 mm from the portal, 4.8 mm to the small saphenous vein, 6.4 mm to the tibial nerve, 9.6 mm to the posterior tibial artery, 17 mm to the medial calcaneal nerve, and 2.7 mm to the FHL tendon. There was little discrepancy with MRI studies with the exception of the tibial nerve, which could not always be appreciated on MRI.[4]

Balci and colleagues[5] similarly studied cadaveric specimens, placing posteromedial and lateral portals but adjusting the position of the ankle, assessing neutral, 15° of dorsiflexion, and 30° of plantarflexion. In neutral, the anterolateral portal was 6 mm from the sural nerve and 1.6 mm from the peroneals. The distance between the medial portal and the FHL was 2.11 mm and from the tibial artery was 6 mm. With increased dorsiflexion, the distance between the posterior portal and the neurovascular bundle medially increased. This finding may suggest that dorsiflexion of the ankle during portal placement may better protect medial vital structures.[5]

PATHOGENESIS

Although a rare condition, os trigonum syndrome may occur acutely through hyperplantarflexion injury or chronically by repetitive plantarflexion stress moments.[6] As the talus rotates plantarly, the accessory ossicle or prominent lateral talar process is impinged between the calcaneus inferiorly and the tibial plafond superiorly. It must also be appreciated that hyperdorsiflexion of the foot can produce avulsion of the lateral talar process by increased tension to the posterior talofibular ligament.[7] This condition has also been referred to as a Shepherd fracture (**Figs. 2–4**).[8]

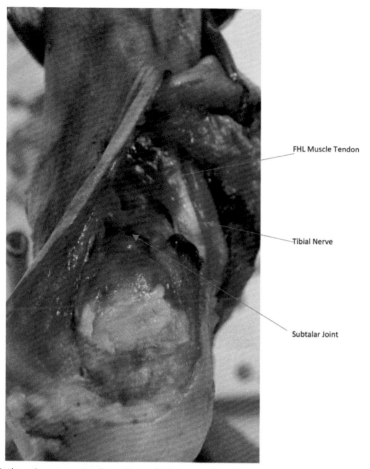

FHL Muscle Tendon

Tibial Nerve

Subtalar Joint

Fig. 1. Cadaveric anatomic dissection of the posterior arthroscopic landmarks. Important anatomic structures medial to the medial portal are the FHL tendon and the tibial nerve. In the center of the working area is the subtalar joint.

In overuse or chronic repetitive plantarflexion injuries, it is thought that the soft tissue is repetitively impinged between the bone entities producing inflammation that gradually results in changes to the adjacent FHL. Recalling the Balci and colleagues[5] study, increased plantarflexion of the ankle produces lateralization of the posterior structures, bringing the FHL tendon into greater risk for impingement. In FHL tenosynovitis, patients may report tenderness in the great toe and posteromedial ankle joint.

PATIENT HISTORY AND PHYSICAL FINDINGS

Appropriate history and physical is obtained to establish the nature, location, onset, duration, and aggravating and mitigating influences of the clinical complaint. Understanding the activities of the individual is also important. In the acute injury, a forced hyperplantarflexion is usually described. In chronic cases of overuse and os trigonum syndrome, pain is frequently noted to the posterolateral aspect of the ankle but can also be seen posteromedial and diffusely to the posterior aspect of the ankle joint.

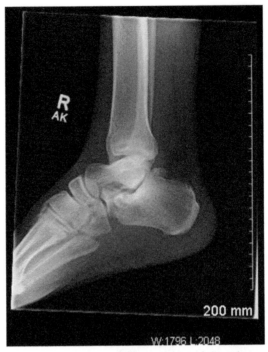

Fig. 2. Radiograph of a fracture of the posterior process of the talus.

During the physical examination, palpation across the posterolateral ankle joint is critical to establish trigger point tenderness. There may be focal swelling in this region. Forced plantarflexion of the foot can reproduce impingement and pain to the area, known as the nutcracker sign.[9]

There may be a decrease in ankle range of motion, particularly in plantarflexion. In chronic cases in which the FHL becomes inflamed, reduction of hallux motion can occur secondary to fibrosis. A provocative maneuver for pain reproduction can be done with the knee in extension, dorsiflexion of the ankle, and attempted hallux dorsiflexion.

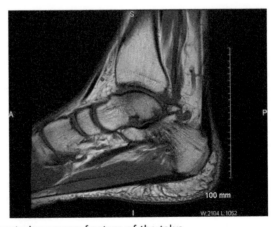

Fig. 3. MRI of a posterior process fracture of the talus.

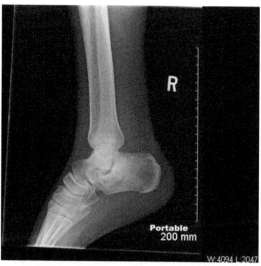

Fig. 4. Plantar flexed radiograph after excision of the posterior process talar fracture.

Diagnostic injections of local anesthetic with image guidance such as fluoroscopy or ultrasonography can help confirm diagnosis if pain relief is achieved with use (**Fig. 5**).

Differential diagnosis based on these findings can include a host of conditions to include fractures of the posterior tibiotalocalcaneal complex, osteochondral lesions

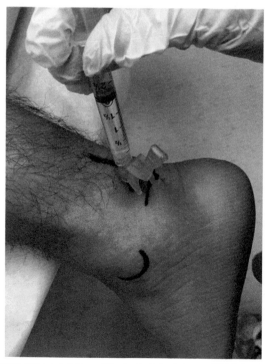

Fig. 5. A diagnostic injection consisting of 2 mL of a 1:1 mixture of 2% lidocaine and 4 mg of Decadron is injected into the flexor tendon sheath through the posterior lateral arthroscopic portal.

of the talus and/or tibia, tarsal coalition, soft tissue lesions, and tendon disorders inclusive of the peroneals and Achilles.

IMAGING

Lateral plain film radiographs are usually adequate to identify the presence of posterolateral talar prominence or an accessory ossicle. Lateral foot plantarflexion images can show posterior impingement on the distal tibia (see **Figs. 2–4**).

Advanced imaging with computed tomography (CT) and MRI can be used if necessary. CT scans can more accurately establish the relationship of bone structures producing the image. They can also benefit the identification of fracture. MRI can identify marrow edema, fluid collections, and most importantly concomitant synovitis of the FHL tendon (**Fig. 6**). Sonography can dynamically examine the gliding of the FHL tendon during passive dorsiflexing and plantarflexing of the ankle.

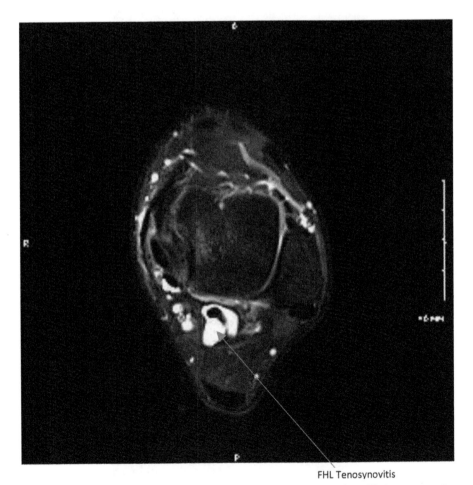

FHL Tenosynovitis

Fig. 6. T2 MRI showing hyperintensity surrounding the FHL tendon, likely representing pathologic tenosynovitis.

TREATMENT

As in any inflammatory process producing local pain and dysfunction, initial nonoperative care includes rest, ice, antiinflammatory medication, and avoidance of activities that exacerbate the condition. A period of immobilization in a walking boot can be considered. Physical therapy to assist in reduction of inflammation may be instituted with progressive range of motion, strengthening, and reconditioning to sport-specific activity. As previously discussed, diagnostic and therapeutic injections of local anesthesia can be administered (see **Fig. 5**). If a corticosteroid is used, it should be done with caution to avoid injecting intratendinously. Image guidance using fluoroscopy or ultrasonography can aid with administration. These injections can assist in understanding the response to surgical intervention if considered.

Failure to respond to nonoperative care for a period of 3 to 6 months suggests that operative intervention may be an acceptable alternative. Older literature presents an open technique both through a posteromedial and posterolateral approach.[10] With advancement of endoscopic technique, much of recent literature is devoted to this approach.

SURGICAL TECHNIQUE

Historically, posterior ankle arthroscopy and/or endoscopy was considered potentially dangerous because of the proximity of vital neurovascular structures.[11] In 2000, van Dijk and colleagues[12] published their approach to posterior ankle arthroendoscopy, creating a method that carefully and systematically avoided the neurovascular bundle. Since that time, posterior impingement treated surgically by an endoscopic approach has been performed more consistently.

Once the patient has completed a 3-month to 6-month course of failed conservative treatment, surgical intervention may be indicated. A thorough preoperative medical work-up should be completed to clear the patient for elective surgery. It is important to take into consideration that the patient will be positioned prone when reviewing pertinent medical history.

POSITIONING

The patient is placed prone on the operating room table with a well-padded thigh or high calf tourniquet. The operative limb is elevated on several blankets, a pillow, or a ramp to raise the affected extremity above the contralateral foot (**Fig. 7**). This

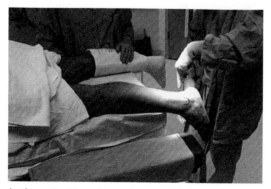

Fig. 7. Preoperatively, the patient is positioned prone with the operative extremity raised above the contralateral limb. Anatomic landmarks are drawn to allow appropriate portal placement.

elevation prevents restriction of movement for the arthroscopic equipment during the procedure. The pelvis should be bumped accordingly to allow the foot to be positioned perpendicular to the floor with the foot resting in a neutral 90° with respect to the leg. Anatomic structures are then drawn out. From the tip of the fibula, a line parallel with the plantar foot is drawn to the medial side. The medial and lateral borders of the Achilles tendon are then marked. The medial and lateral portals are drawn just above the intersection where the medial and lateral borders of the Achilles tendon meet the transverse line. A line is then drawn across the bottom of the foot extending from the lateral portal to the first web space (**Figs. 8** and **9**).[12–16]

TECHNIQUE

The extremity is then scrubbed, prepped, and draped with aseptic technique. The skin overlying the lateral portal is sharply created with care to not penetrate through subcutaneous tissue. Blunt dissection using a mosquito hemostat is taken down to the level of bone in the same direction as the line drawn to the first web space. The hemostat is then replaced for a 30° 4.0 mm endoscope with saline set to gravity (Video 1). The medial portal is then created just medial to the Achilles tendon in the same plane as the lateral portal. A hemostat is inserted through the portal at 90° to the scope just deep to the Achilles tendon. The scope is held pointing to the first web space and is used as a guide for the hemostat to travel down to the level of bone, thereby avoiding the neurovascular bundle. The hemostat is then replaced with a shaver. To obtain a visual of the surrounding structures, some of the fat surrounding the scope must be excised.[12–16]

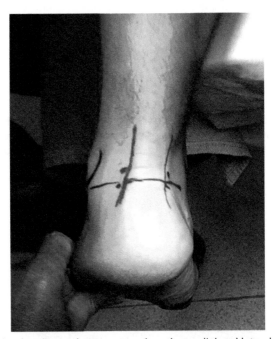

Fig. 8. Anatomic landmarks are drawn out to place the medial and lateral posterior portals. A parallel line is drawn horizontally across the posterior ankle starting at the posterior tip of the fibula. The portals are drawn just medial and lateral to the level of the Achilles just above the horizontal joint line.

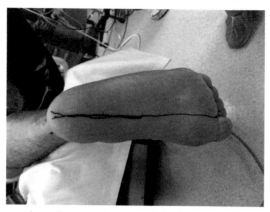

Fig. 9. A line is drawn along the second ray to guide alignment of the posterior scope during the procedure. This line helps prevent invasion of the medial neurovascular structures.

Anatomic landmarks and disorders can then be evaluated. The FHL tendon is medial to the Stieda process along the posterior joint capsule. It is important to identify the FHL tendon and work laterally to avoid compromise of the neurovascular structures.

Flexion and extension of the toe aid in this visualization. Ligamentous structures, including the posterior inferior tibiofibular ligament, posterior talofibular ligament, and calcaneofibular ligament, should be visible lateral to the FHL. Deep to the capsule, the posterior aspects of the subtalar and ankle joints can be inspected. These structures are flanked laterally by the fibula and peroneal tendons and medially by the FHL tendon, the neurovascular bundle, the flexor digitorum longus, posterior tibial tendon, and the medial malleolus.[16]

Many disorders can be addressed using this technique, such as posterior ankle and subtalar joint osteochondral lesions, subtalar/ankle arthritis, soft tissue impingement, bony impingement, arthroscopic evaluation of fracture reduction, FHL or peroneal tenosynovitis, and excision of talocalcaneal coalitions (Video 2).[16] The portals can then be closed primarily with application of a soft dressing, splint, or cast (**Fig. 10**).

Alternatively, Horibe and colleagues[17] described a different method for excision of a symptomatic os trigonum. They proposed using the posterolateral portal as described by van Dijk and colleagues,[12] but instead of the typical posterior medial portal they used an accessory posterolateral portal. In the transverse plane, this portal was placed just below the fibular tip and posterior to the peroneal tendons.

REHABILITATION AND RECOVERY

The postoperative protocol differs with each type of procedure. van Dijk and colleagues[12] placed a soft postoperative dressing after a symptomatic os trigonum excision in a ballet dancer. The patient was then instructed to perform ankle joint range of motion exercises starting immediately after surgery followed by weight bearing after 3 days. Physical therapy was initiated 2 weeks postoperatively and the patient returned to professional dancing after 6 weeks.[12] Gasparetto and colleagues[13] recommended weight bearing to tolerance for patients who underwent an FHL release, posterior impingement release, and osteochondral lesion debridement. After posterior impingement release, Miyamoto and colleagues[14] placed a soft dressing and allowed partial weight bearing to tolerance on postoperative day 1. Full weight bearing was

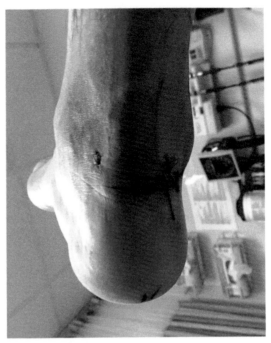

Fig. 10. Primary closure of the posterior arthroscopic portals.

permitted according to pain tolerance, and return to activity was allowed when the patient was able to perform full range of motion to the affected foot. A review by Kerkhoffs and colleagues[11] suggested a compressive dressing and partial weight bearing for 3 to 5 days with active range of motion for surgical posterior impingement release. Physical therapy may or may not be indicated. The athlete was expected to return to sport at 6 to 8 weeks.[11]

CLINICAL RESULTS IN THE LITERATURE

In van Dijk and colleagues'[12] original article from 2000, they presented a case study of a professional ballet dancer who returned to dancing 6 weeks after the surgery. At 30 months, she had no complaints, no recurrence of symptoms, and was professionally dancing. He reported that between 1995 and the publication of the article in 2000, 86 endoscopic hindfoot procedures were performed without complications.[12]

In 2016, Spennacchio and colleagues[18] performed a systematic review of the literature regarding all studies reporting posterior ankle endoscopy. The studies were evaluated and categorized by level of evidence. They were also categorized based on whether the literature was for, against, or had conflicting findings regarding the indication for posterior endoscopy. The studies were reviewed by 2 independent researchers. Out of 46 articles and 766 procedures, there were no studies with level I or level II evidence. Nine studies reported American Orthopaedic Foot and Ankle Society (AOFAS) scores and found the cumulative increase to be 2389 points. They found an overall minor complication rate of less than 7% and major complication rate of less than 2%. They concluded that the literature was in favor of performing an endoscopic approach for posterior ankle impingement.[18]

Zwiers and colleagues[19] performed a systematic review of the literature in 2013 comparing open and endoscopic treatment of posterior ankle impingement. Sixteen articles were analyzed for the study based on inclusion criteria and exclusion criteria. Out of the accepted 16 studies, 419 ankles were treated. For the open technique, 145 procedures were performed, with 2 studies using a lateral approach, 2 using a medial, and 2 using both medial and lateral. In 3 studies, patient satisfaction was reported as excellent or good in 85.1% of cases. In 2 studies, AOFAS scores were weighted post-operatively to 90.5 points. Three studies reported a return to activity in 7 to 20 weeks with a weighted average of 16 weeks. Complications were recorded in total at 15.9% with 2.1% considered major and 13.8% minor. In comparison, 274 endoscopic proce-dures were performed with the standard 2-portal incisions. In 3 studies, the patient satisfaction was reported as excellent or good in 80.9% of cases. Seven studies re-ported AOFAS scores with a weighted mean of 91.3 points postoperatively. Four studies reported a return to activity with a weighted average of 11.3 weeks. Compli-cations were recorded in all studies with 1.8% considered major and 5.4% minor. The investigators suggested that the level of evidence is limited and that obtaining high-quality evidence is important. Overall, the findings theorize that both the open and endoscopic approaches have good outcomes. However, the investigators sug-gested that an endoscopic approach should be considered based on the lower rates of complications and shorter time to return to full activity.[19]

Ribbans and colleagues[10] performed a literature review to determine the efficacy of conservative, open, and endoscopic treatment of posterior impingement syndrome. Forty-seven articles fitted the inclusion and exclusion criteria. The level of evidence did not exceed level IV (case report/case series) or level V (expert opinion). Conservative treatment of posterior impingement syndrome included rest, cessation of activity, technique modification, physical therapy, orthotics, nonsteroidal antiin-flammatory drugs, and injections. The review of the literature found little information beyond an article in 1997 recommending conservative treatment but not commenting on efficacy. Two small case series studies suggested curative outcomes with ultrasonography-guided posterior corticosteroid injections. With open surgical inter-vention, 357 operations were reviewed. The overall complication rate was 3.9% to 7% for medial approaches and 14.7% for lateral incisions. The overall nerve injury rate was 4.2% with a lower incidence with a medial approach. Using an endoscopic approach, 521 procedures were analyzed. The posterior medial and posterolateral portals described by van Dijk and colleagues[12] were used in 77.2% of the cases. The overall complication rate was 4.8% with a nerve injury complication rate of 3.7%. No difference was found comparing open versus endoscopic procedures. The investigators expressed difficulty in comparing the two procedures because of a lack of standardized outcomes. They concluded that a more precise indicator was the return to sport time. In 249 open procedures, 73% of the patients were involved in an activity and averaged a return to sport in 14.8 weeks. In the arthroen-doscopic group, 67% of 326 patients were involved in sports and averaged a return to sport in 8.9 weeks. Overall there seems to be a quicker return to sport in the arthroendoscopic group, but the investigators stressed the lack of consistent data to compare the different approaches.[12]

Nickisch and colleagues[20] performed a scientific review in 2012 of 189 hindfoot arthroscopic procedure complications from 2001 to 2009 at 2 universities. The surgeries were performed by 6 different surgeons and there was a mean follow-up of 17 months. They did note that 40.3% of patients did not have a follow-up past 12 months. Out of 189 procedures, 60.8% were intra-articular, including subtalar debridement, subtalar fusion, ankle debridement, osteochondral defect repair, partial talectomy, fixation of calcaneal fractures, and revision of subtalar nonunion. Extra-articular disorders consisted of 27% of the procedures, which included excision of os trigonum, tenolysis of FHL tendon, and partial calcanectomy. For the extra-articular procedures, the arthroscope was introduced as described by van Dijk and colleagues.[12] The overall complication rate was 8.5%. Of 16 patients with complications, 7 were neurologic. Four patients had plantar numbness and 3 completely resolved. Three patients experienced sural nerve dysesthesia and 2 resolved. Postoperative infections were seen in 2 patients. One infection required intravenous antibiotics and the other required surgical incision and drainage. Both patients had resolution. Complex regional pain syndrome was seen in 2 patients, who were successfully treated with a multidisciplinary approach of physical therapy, medications, and local anesthetic blocks. Postoperative posterior muscular tightness was seen in 4 patients, 3 of whom had undergone extra-articular procedures. All were treated with physiotherapy and had resolution of symptoms. There were differences in complication rates between the surgeons with more experience versus those with less experience. Of the 7 patients with nerve-related complications, 2 underwent complex reconstruction including arthroscopic debridement of the ankle and subtalar joints, 2 had a lateral accessory portal placed for a subtalar joint fusion, 1 had an excision of an os trigonum, and 1 had tenolysis of the FHL tendon. Overall, no statistical significance was found for neurologic complications with patients more than 50 years old, female sex, surgeon inexperience, posterior endoscopic procedures, operative time more than 120 minutes, distraction, tourniquet use, and tourniquet use more than 90 minutes. The investigators acknowledged that further research is warranted because theirs was retrospective, involved several surgeons, and had a high variability in procedures. Overall, the investigators showed that posterior arthroscopy and endoscopy can be safely performed with a low rate of postoperative complications.[20]

In summary there is sufficient level IV and V evidence reporting good outcomes and low complication rates with posterior arthroendoscopy for treatment of posterior impingement syndrome; however, it is evident that there is a need for better-quality evidence with a more standardized reporting of outcomes and complications.

SUPPLEMENTARY DATA

Supplementary data related to this article can be found at http://dx.doi.org/10.1016/j.cpm.2016.06.009.

REFERENCES

1. Grogan DP, Walling AK, Ogden JA. Anatomy of the os trigonum. J Pediatr Orthop 1990;10:618–22.
2. Steida, L. 1869. Ueber secundare fusswurselkochen. Archiv Fur Anatomie, Physiologie, under Wissenshcaftliche Medicine, 108.
3. Mann RW, Osley DW. Os trigonum. Variation of a common accessory ossicle of the talus. J Am Podiatr Med Assoc 1990;80:536–9.
4. Sitler DF, Amendola A, Bailey CS, et al. Posterior ankle arthroscopy: an anatomic study. J Bone Joint Surg Am 2002;84(5):763–9.
5. Balci HI, Polat G, Dikmen G, et al. Safety of posterior ankle arthroscopy portals in different ankle positions: a cadaveric study. Knee Surg Sports Traumatol Arthrosc 2016;24(7):2119–23.
6. Nault ML, Kocher MS, Micheli LJ. Os trigonum syndrome. J Am Acad Orthop Surg 2014;22:545–53.
7. Hedrick MR, McBryde AM. Posterior ankle impingement. Foot Ankle Int 1994;15:2–8.

8. Shepherd FJ. A hitherto undescribed fracture of the astragalus. J Anat Physiol 1882;17:79–81.
9. Schubert JC, Adler DC. Talar fractures. In: Banks AS, Downey MS, Martin DE, editors. McGlamry's comprehensive book of foot and ankle surgery, vol. 1, 3rd edition. Philadelphia: Lippincott Williams & Wilkins; 2001. p. 1871–4.
10. Ribbans WJ, Ribbans HA, Cruickshank JA, et al. The management of posterior ankle impingement syndrome in sport: a review. Foot Ankle Surg 2015;21:1–10.
11. Kerkhoffs GM, de Leeuw PA, d'Hooghe PP. Posterior ankle impingement. In: d'Hooghe P, Kerkhoffs G, editors. The ankle in football. Paris: Springer; 2014. p. 141–54.
12. van Dijk CN, Scholten PE, Krips R. A 2-portal endoscopic approach for diagnosis and treatment of posterior ankle pathology. Arthroscopy 2000;16(8):871–6.
13. Gasparetto F, Collo G, Pisanu G, et al. Posterior ankle and subtalar arthroscopy: indications, technique, and results. Curr Rev Musculoskelet Med 2012;5(2): 164–70.
14. Miyamoto W, Takao M, Matsushita T. Hindfoot endoscopy for posterior ankle impingement syndrome and flexor hallucis longus tendon disorders. Foot Ankle Clin 2015;20(1):139–47.
15. Lijoi F, Lughi M, Baccarani G. Posterior arthroscopic approach to the ankle. Arthroscopy 2003;19(1):62–7.
16. Smyth NA, Zwiers R, Wiegerinck JI, et al. Posterior hindfoot arthroscopy a review. Am J Sports Med 2014;42(1):225–34.
17. Horibe S, Kita K, Natsu-ume T, et al. A novel technique of arthroscopic excision of a symptomatic os trigonum. Arthroscopy 2008;24(1):121.e1-4.
18. Spennacchio P, Cucchi D, Randelli PS, et al. Evidence-based indications for hindfoot endoscopy. Knee Surg Sports Traumatol Arthrosc 2016;24(4):1386–95.
19. Zwiers R, Wiegerinck JI, Murawski CD, et al. Surgical treatment for posterior ankle impingement. Arthroscopy 2013;29(7):1263–70.
20. Nickisch F, Barg A, Saltzman CL, et al. Postoperative complications of posterior ankle and hindfoot arthroscopy. J Bone Joint Surg Am 2012;94(5):439–46.

Endoscopic Plantar Fascia Debridement for Chronic Plantar Fasciitis

 CrossMark

James M. Cottom, DPM*, Joseph S. Baker, DPM, AACFAS

KEYWORDS

- Heel pain • Plantar fasciitis • Endoscopic • Debridement

KEY POINTS

- When conservative therapy fails for chronic plantar fasciitis, surgical intervention may be an option.
- Surgical techniques that maintain the integrity of the plantar fascia will have less risk of destabilizing the foot and will retain foot function.
- Endoscopic debridement of the plantar fascia can be performed reproducibly to reduce pain and maintain function of the foot.

Plantar heel pain is one of the most common conditions seen in the clinics of foot and ankle surgeons. Approximately 10% of the general population will experience heel pain in the form of plantar fasciitis at least once in their lifetime.[1–4] The most commonly cited cause of plantar fasciitis is the pull of the proximal insertion of the plantar fascia on the calcaneus.[5–8] The plantar fascia serves an important role in the gait cycle, because it helps to support the arch of the foot as well as aids in resupination of the foot during propulsion.[1,9,10]

When conservative treatment of chronic plantar fasciitis is not successful, surgical intervention may become an option. A popular method of addressing this chronic condition is to perform a plantar fasciotomy, whereby the medial one-third to one-half of the plantar fascia is transected.[11] However, different investigators have shown that a plantar fasciotomy is not performed without consequence. Daly and colleagues[12] found a significant decrease in the height of the longitudinal arch as well a less efficient gait in patients who had undergone plantar fasciotomy versus a control. A cadaveric study performed by Ward and colleagues[13] showed that as the plantar fascia was released sequentially from medial to lateral, the force increased on the remaining lateral fibers, and the subtalar joint lost its ability to resupinate.

Florida Orthopedic Foot and Ankle Center, 2030 Bee Ridge Road, Suite C, Sarasota, FL 34239, USA
* Corresponding author.
E-mail address: jamescottom300@hotmail.com

Clin Podiatr Med Surg 33 (2016) 545–551
http://dx.doi.org/10.1016/j.cpm.2016.06.004
0891-8422/16/$ – see front matter © 2016 Elsevier Inc. All rights reserved.

podiatric.theclinics.com

In light of these findings, the authors propose an innovative technique to address chronic plantar fasciitis surgically, without disrupting the integrity of the plantar fascia. This technique was introduced to the senior author (J.M.C.) (K Bramlett, MD, personal communication, 2011).

OPERATIVE TECHNIQUE

The patient is first given a popliteal nerve block in the preoperative holding area and is then brought in to the operating room. The patient is then placed supine on the operating table with the operative extremity in external rotation, so that the lateral border of the foot is allowed to lay flat against the table. A bump placed under the contralateral hip can be used to assist in positioning when necessary. Following exsanguination of the extremity, a thigh tourniquet is then inflated to 300 mm Hg. Using a surgical marker, the medial malleolus is then outlined, and a straight line is drawn from the posterior aspect of the medial malleolus to the heel. The first portal is marked out along this line at or slightly above the level of the plantar fascia. The second portal is then placed 2 cm distal to the first portal at or slightly above the level of the plantar fascia (**Fig. 1**). The intention is to enter the space directly superior to the plantar fascia, so it is helpful to place the portals slightly superior to the plantar fascia.

Full-thickness incisions can then be made with a number 11 blade at the portal sites. A curved hemostat is used for blunt dissection and to identify the plantar fascia. A 4.0-mm camera can then be placed into the distal portal, while a 3.5-mm shaver is introduced into the proximal portal (**Fig. 2**). A spinal needle is then inserted from the plantar fell into the most painful area, which should be identified preoperatively. This technique allows for direct visualization and debridement of the most painful part of the plantar fascia. This technique can also be used to orient the surgeon during the procedure, because bony landmarks are scarce. Debridement of inflammatory tissue along the superior aspect of the plantar fascia can then be debrided using the arthroscopic shaver under direct visualization (**Fig. 3**). The calcaneal spur can then be identified and removed as necessary (**Fig. 4**). Removal of the spur can then be confirmed with intraoperative fluoroscopy (**Fig. 5**). The plantar fascia can be thinned out with a

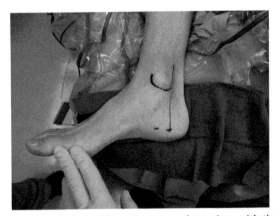

Fig. 1. The operative extremity is positioned in external rotation, with the lateral border of the foot against the operating room table. The medial malleolus is traced, and a line is drawn along its posterior border. The proximal portal is established slightly superior to the level of the plantar fascia. The distal portal is established at the same level, 2 cm distal to the first portal.

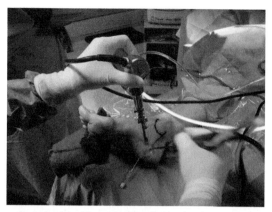

Fig. 2. The 4.0-mm camera is placed into the distal portal, whereas a 3.5-mm shaver is placed into the proximal portal. Note that an 18-gauge spinal needle has been introduced through the plantar foot in the area of maximal tenderness. This assists the surgeon in orientation during the procedure.

shaver or with an ablator to estimate physiologic thickness (**Fig. 6**). An arthroscopic probe is then used to confirm that the plantar fascia is intact, and that the integrity of the structure has not been compromised (**Fig. 7**). Once the surgeon is satisfied, the instrumentation can be removed, and the portal sites can be closed with 3-0 nylon suture (**Fig. 8**).

In the senior author's practice, patients are allowed to bear weight on the operative extremity in a removable, below-the-knee, adjustable immobilization boot postoperatively. Physical therapy is typically initiated after 3 weeks, and patients are allowed to return to their normal shoes after 4 weeks.

RESULTS

This procedure has been performed on a series of 46 patients, who were followed up for a mean of 20.51 months. Mean patient age in this group was 52.8 ± 13.67 years

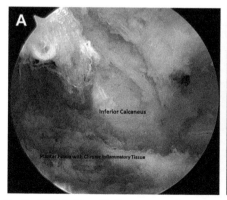
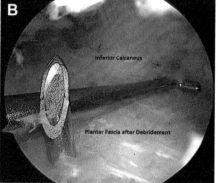

Fig. 3. (*A*) Bright red inflammatory tissue noted along the superior aspect of the plantar fascia. (*B*) After initial debridement of the inflammatory tissue, the plantar fascia is identified. Note the tip of the arthroscopic probe is between the inferior aspect of the calcaneus and the plantar fascia origin.

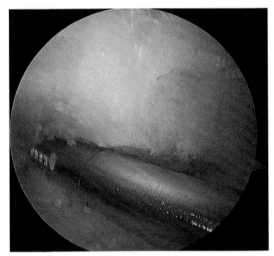

Fig. 4. The arthroscopic shaver can be placed in the interval between the superior plantar fascia and the inferior calcaneus, and the exostosis can be removed.

old. The mean duration of conservative treatment before the index operation was 33.07 ± 37.49 months. The visual analogue scores in this patient group improved from 8.95 ± 1.41 preoperatively to 1.34 ± 1.25 postoperatively. The complication rate was low, with 6 cases (13%) of paresthesia along the plantar foot, all of which resolved without intervention within 10 months. There were also 3 patients (6.5%) who had delayed healing of a portal site, all of which were treated successfully with local wound care and oral antibiotics.

DISCUSSION

Chronic plantar fasciitis that does not respond to conservative treatment can be frustrating for the patient as well as the provider. There are several surgical options for treatment, but there is still not a consensus on the ideal surgical procedure.[14] Plantar fascia release remains a popular option, although it has been scrutinized for its potential complications. Brugh and colleagues[15] performed a prospective study reviewing the amount of the plantar fascia released and the association with lateral column

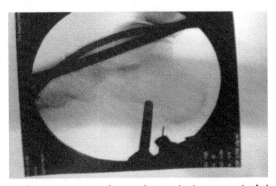

Fig. 5. Intraoperative fluoroscopy may be used to assist in removal of the spur.

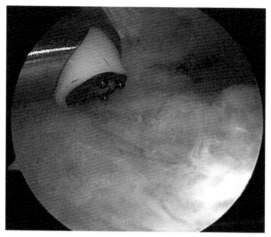

Fig. 6. An arthroscopic ablator can be used to thin out the plantar fascia to its physiologic thickness.

pain. Although all of the patients were reported to have decreased heel pain following the procedure, pain along the lateral column increased significantly when more than 50% of the plantar fascia was released. Lundeen and colleagues[16] examined 53 patients who had undergone endoscopic plantar fasciotomy. Although they reported a satisfaction rate of 81.1%, the unsatisfied group complained of metatarsalgia 50% of the time. Patients also reported continued pain in the arch of the foot.

With this information in mind, the authors present an innovative surgical approach to plantar fasciitis, which does not compromise the integrity of the plantar fascia insertion into the calcaneus. The technique has been shown to be effective at reducing pain in a series of patients. This technique also allows for endoscopic excision of a concomitant infracalcaneal exostosis when necessary.

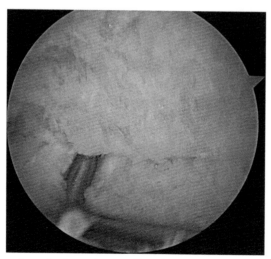

Fig. 7. An arthroscopic probe is used to confirm the attachment of the plantar fascia remains after debridement.

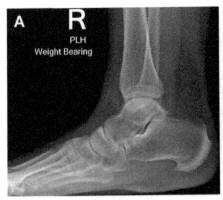 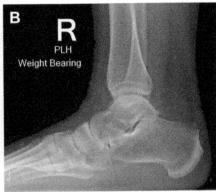

Fig. 8. Preoperative (*A*) and postoperative (*B*) lateral radiographs of a patient who underwent endoscopic plantar fascia debridement with infracalcaneal exostosis excision.

REFERENCES

1. Uden H, Boesch E, Kumar S, et al. Plantar fasciitis—to jab or to support? A systematic review of the current best evidence. J Multidiscip Healthc 2011;4:155–64.
2. Roos EM, Engstrom M, Soderberg B. Foot orthoses for the treatment of plantar fasciitis. Foot Ankle Int 2006;27:606–11.
3. Landorf KB, Keenan AM, Herbert RD. Effectiveness of different types of foot orthoses for the treatment of plantar fasciitis. J Am Podiatr Med Assoc 2004;94:542–9.
4. Seligman DA, Dawson DR. Customized heel pads and soft orthotics to treat heel pain and plantar fasciitis. Arch Phys Med Rehabil 2003;84:1564–7.
5. Thomas JL, Christensen JC, Kravitz SR, et al. The diagnosis and treatment of heel pain: a clinical practice guideline—revision 2010. J Foot Ankle Surg 2010;49:S1–19.
6. Bergmann JN. History and mechanical control of heel spur pain. Clin Podiatr Med Surg 1990;7:243–59.
7. McCarthy DJ, Gorecki GE. The anatomical basis of inferior calcaneal lesions. J Am Podiatr Med Assoc 1979;69:527–36.
8. Fuller EA. The windlass mechanism of the foot. A mechanical model to explain pathology. J Am Podiatr Med Assoc 2000;90:35–46.
9. Michaud TC. Foot orthoses and other forms of conservative foot care. Newton (MA): Lippincott, Williams & Wilkins; 1997.
10. Lisowski FP. A guide to dissection of the human body. 2nd edition. Singapore: World Scientific Publishing Company; 2004.
11. Boberg JS, Dauphinée DM, Malay DS, et al. Plantar heel. In: Southerland JT, editor. McGlamry's comprehensive textbook of foot and ankle surgery. 4th edition. Philadelphia: Lippincott Williams & Wilkins; 2013. p. 1586–624.
12. Daly PJ, Kitaoka HB, Chao EYS. Plantar fasciotomy for intractable plantar fasciitis: clinical results and biomechanical evaluation. Foot Ankle 1992;13:188.
13. Ward ED, Smith KM, Cocheba JR, et al. In vivo forces in the plantar fascia during the stance phase of gait. J Am Podiatr Med Assoc 2003;93:429–42.
14. DiGiovanni BF, Moore AM, Zlotnicki JP, et al. Preferred management of recalcitrant plantar fasciitis among orthopaedic foot and ankle surgeons. Foot Ankle Int 2012;33:507–12.

15. Brugh AM, Fallat LM, Savoy-Moore RT. Lateral column symptomatology following plantar fascial release: a prospective study. J Foot Ankle Surg 2002;41:365–71.
16. Lundeen RO, Aziz S, Burks JB, et al. Endoscopic plantar fasciotomy: a retrospective analysis of results in 53 patients. J Foot Ankle Surg 2000;39:208–17.

Arthroscopic Repair of Ankle Instability

Matthew D. Sorensen, DPM*, John Baca, DPM, Keith Arbuckle, DPM[1]

KEYWORDS

- Arthroscopy • Broström • Lateral ankle • Ankle stabilization

KEY POINTS

- Arthroscopic parameters and indications continue to expand as technological advances and scientific understanding of biomechanical pathology in the foot and ankle continue to improve.
- Additionally, understanding of the proprioceptive contribution to an unstable ankle joint has opened up less-invasive approaches to surgical intervention in the ankle.
- Minimally invasive approaches have a proven benefit of decreased soft-tissue plane dissection, decreased overall soft-tissue embarrassment, and subsequent decreased fibrotic scar tissue deposition tendency postoperatively.
- Lower-profile scars involved in arthroscopic approaches decrease the need for prolonged immobilization, allowing for earlier and safe joint mobilization. Secondary to these perceived and apparent benefits, there is capacity to significantly improve patient outcomes in the active population perioperatively and in the long term.
- A strong understanding of topographic anatomy, natural history and pathobiomechanics, and experienced arthroscopic skills are necessary to mitigate risk profiles in arthroscopic approaches to surgical intervention in chronic lateral ankle instability.

INTRODUCTION

Ankle sprains are a common injury among athletic and non-athletic individuals, at an annual rate of over 3 million injuries per year in the United States.[1] Ankle sprains make up 10% of visits to the emergency department, with 30,000 visits occurring per day.[2] Most sprains are the result of athletic activity in a younger population, with basketball being the cause of 41% of athletically related sprains.[1]

Although most sprains heal uneventfully, about 20% of patients will develop chronic ankle instability after a sprain.[3,4] Ankle instability is characterized by recurrent sprains, difficulty with ambulation on uneven ground, and sometimes pain with activity.[3,5,6]

Disclosure Statement: consultant and design surgeon, Stryker Orthopedics; consultant, Treace Medical Concepts; consultant and design surgeon, Trilliant (M.D. Sorensen).
Weil Foot & Ankle Institute, Chicago, IL, USA
[1] Present address: 1132 Cove Drive, Prospect Heights, IL 60070.
* Corresponding author. Weil Foot & Ankle Institute, 1455 East Golf Road, Des Plaines, IL 60016.
E-mail address: mdsoren34@gmail.com

Clin Podiatr Med Surg 33 (2016) 553–564
http://dx.doi.org/10.1016/j.cpm.2016.06.010
0891-8422/16/© 2016 Elsevier Inc. All rights reserved.

podiatric.theclinics.com

The diagnosis of ankle instability is based on history, clinical examination, and radiographs.[7] It is important to avoid undertreatment of chronic ankle instability, as it may lead to early degeneration of the ankle due to unbalanced loading of the medial ankle.[7]

INJURY AND ANATOMY OF THE LIGAMENTS

The mechanism of injury is usually a forced adduction and inversion of the foot while the ankle is plantarflexed.[8] In this position, the anterior talofibular ligament (ATFL) is taut, and the ankle is less stable due the decrease in width of the posterior articular surface of the talus.[3,9] The ATFL is the most commonly injured ligament out of the lateral ankle ligament complex.[9,10] The calcaneofibular ligament (CFL) and the posterior talofibular ligament (PTFL) can also be injured, but these are not as frequent as an ATFL injury.

The surgeon must understand the ligamentous anatomy in order to properly restore ankle function. The ATFL is the main lateral stabilizer of the ankle joint and originates 1 cm proximal to the tip of the fibula.[11] This ligament is 7.2 mm wide, intracapsular, most often consists 2 bands, and inserts just distal to the articular surface of the talus and 18 mm superior to the subtalar joint.[9,12] The origin of the CFL is 8 mm above the tip of the fibula. The CFL the courses posterior to the fibula, under the peroneal tendons, and inserts on the calcaneus 13 mm distal to the subtalar joint.[3] The angle formed by the ATFL and the CFL is 121°.[11]

TREATMENT

Conservative therapy initially entails rest, ice, compression, and elevation.[3] Rehabilitation strategies should include peroneal muscle strengthening, proprioceptive training, and bracing.[3,13,14] External bracing is a viable option to help add extrinsic stability to the ankle joint in addition to aiding the cerebral awareness of the ankle position proprioceptively. For some patients, however, this may not add adequate stability, or they may be unable to tolerate this device as a definitive solution.[15] Surgical repair becomes a necessary and viable option for this group of patients. Those with continued chronic ankle instability, despite appropriate and deliberate conservative intervention, may also become candidates for surgery. Often an MRI (**Fig. 1**) is obtained to evaluate the lateral ankle ligament complex and evaluate for associated injuries including those to the talar dome and peroneal tendons, further enhancing and directing definitive treatment.[13]

HISTORY OF STABILIZATION PROCEDURES

More than 50 procedures have been described for repair of lateral ankle ligaments.[14] Traditionally these procedures fall into 2 reconstructive categories; anatomic and nonanatomic/augmented.[16] Anatomic repair seeks to repair injured ligaments primarily or with local tissue that maintains motion without sacrificing subtalar joint motion. This will allow for physiologic inhibition of anterior translation, axial plane rotation, and inversion of the talus within the mortise without blocking subtalar and ankle motion.[14]

Nonanatomic reconstruction does not restore local anatomy, and is used to create robust restraint to abnormal motion of the ankle joint.[17] Commonly used nonanatomic reconstructive procedures are modifications of those described by Watson-Jones,[18] Chrisman and Snook,[19] and Evans.[20] These repairs have been shown to alter the biomechanics and loading of the hindfoot, midfoot, and forefoot.[21–23]

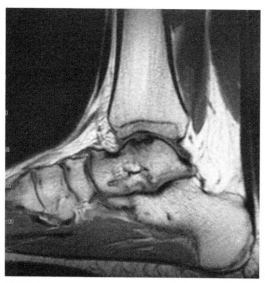

Fig. 1. T1 weighted MRI demonstrating osteochondral defect of the talar dome.

The open modified Broström is an anatomic repair that is accepted as the reference standard for lateral ankle ligament repair.[4,16,20,24] The Broström consists of imbrication of the ATFL and joint capsule.[16] This was described by Broström in 1966, then modified later by Gould,[25] who added reinforcement of the repair with the interior extensor retinaculum. The Broström-Gould technique has been shown to restore proper ankle kinematics and reduce the risk of degenerative ankle arthritis.[4,16,18,26]

NEED FOR ARTHROSCOPY

Lateral ankle stabilization procedures have had high success rates on the order of 80% to 95% toward restoring predictable ankle stability and function.[17,27] Despite these encouragingly high success rates, 13% to 35% of patients may continue to experience symptoms after surgery.[28,29] Isolated chondral injury is not always detectable with preoperative MRI. Komenda and Ferkel showed that 96% of ankles had intra-articular pathology when undergoing arthroscopy prior to lateral ankle stabilization procedures.[23]

The trend of arthroscopic evaluation and debridement followed immediately by open ligament reconstruction mirrors the previous surgical trends of knee and shoulder instability prior to current arthroscopic techniques developed in those joints.[15] Multiple studies have recently shown clinical outcomes to be nearly identical between arthroscopic techniques and open lateral ankle ligament reconstruction.[4,15–20,22–30] When safe zones are identified and maintained intraoperatively, there is minimal risk for neurovascular injury.[18,31] Acevedo found the structure most at risk of injury to be the intermediate branch of the superficial peroneal nerve, which can be found at an average of 20 mm from the medal-most suture.[18] Biomechanical testing has shown equivalent strength and stiffness between arthroscopic lateral ankle stabilization techniques and a traditional open Broström-Gould technique using match-paired cadavers.[32,33] Finally, the arthroscopic Broström technique can help minimize difficulties encountered with traditional open ligament reconstruction. These can include fluid extravasation, which can make normal tissue planes ambiguous, and increased soft tissue swelling and pain, which are often associated with larger open incisions.[15]

Additionally, the arthroscopic approach decreases the level of soft-tissue dissection with subsequent lower levels of tissue plane disruption and effective decrease in scar tissue deposition and decreased soft-tissue impingement pain postoperatively.

Faster Return to Function

With any advancement in surgical approach, one looks for outcome benefit to the patient's endpoint and in decreasing morbidity throughout the perioperative phases of intervention. Karlsson and colleagues[34] noted that athletes undergoing earlier mobilization of the ankle joint after anatomic repair returned to sporting activities quicker and had increased plantar flexion strength compared with those who were immobilized. Cottom and Rigby have allowed patients to bear weight as early as 10 days postoperatively without additional complications and the same outcome.[16] Theoretically, an all-arthroscopic approach allows for a comparatively earlier mobilization over the joint with less concern over adequate time to soft-tissue healing and potential sequalae associated with motion across larger incision sites.

SURGICAL TECHNIQUE
Indications for Surgery

The history and physical examination are key to identifying candidates for the arthroscopic Broström procedure. Patients may relate a history of recurrent lateral ankle sprains or feelings of the ankle giving out, which may or may not improve with external bracing. Although bracing may be helpful in some patients, many are not able to tolerate it on a daily basis. Additionally, and importantly, patients with functional instability may feel continued instability even with the aid of an external sports brace, as the cerebral cortex has lost connection with neuroreceptors within the lateral ankle and cannot identify ankle position in 3-dimensional space.

Patients may often have increased excursion of the talus with anterior drawer and talar tilt manual testing consistent with what is identified as mechanical lateral ankle instability (**Figs. 2** and **3**). Generally, the mechanically unstable ankle has significant and concomitant deficits in proprioceptive capacity of the affected ankle and is why the arthroscopic approach has proven effective even in these scenarios. The authors are finding, and it has been postulated, that the functional component to the unstable ankle is at least as important, if not more important, that the mechanical contribution to instability.

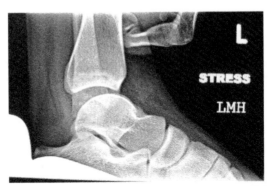

Fig. 2. Radiograph of anterior drawer stress test demonstrating insufficiency of the ATFL.

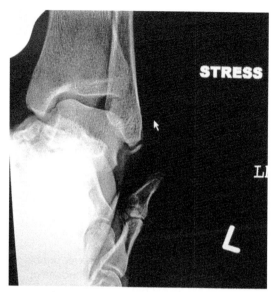

Fig. 3. Inversion stress test demonstrating an insufficient CFL.

It has been stated that surgery should not be considered until failing appropriate conservative intervention, including bracing and physical therapy, which focuses on strengthening and proprioceptive capacities.[27] A modified Rhomberg test is useful to evaluate for functional instability. That said, it is the authors' opinion that conservative intervention should not be palliated unnecessarily for extended periods. The authors use the general guideline of a minimum of 3 months of conservative intervention and maximum of 4 months as the threshold for moving forward surgically when patients do not respond.

Contraindications to the procedure include collagen disorders, hyperelasticity syndromes, and recurrent injury postindex Broström procedure or recurrence after appropriate surgical care. The arthroscopic Broström procedure should also be used judiciously in extremely high physical demand vocations and high-demand laborers as well.[2,3,5,11,12,14,15,21] Patients displaying these contraindications may need consideration for allograft reconstruction techniques.[3,14,15,19,20,23,35,36]

Preparation and Patient Positioning

The arthroscopic lateral ankle stabilization procedure should be performed under general anesthesia or sedation, with concomitant popliteal and saphenous regional nerve block. The patient should be positioned supine on the operating table. A towel bump may be placed beneath the ipsilateral hip to allow for coaxial access to each portal. The authors prefer a noninvasive ankle distractor (**Fig. 4**) in addition to a thigh holder (**Fig. 5**) that is placed during patient positioning. Preoperative identification of anatomic landmarks is essential to avoid injury to at-risk structures. The lateral safe zone includes the anterior distal fibula, the superior margin of the peroneal tendons, and the inferior border of the intermediate branch of the superficial peroneal nerve. The inferior extensor retinaculum (IER) is then marked 1.5 cm from the distal fibula.[18]

Authors' Preferred Method of Procedure

Initially, and once arthroscopic access is gained into the joint, the ankle is addressed in standard fashion to clear and debride apparent synovitic tissue or impingement

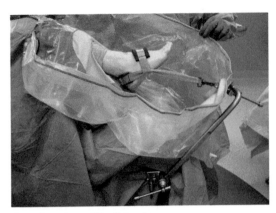

Fig. 4. Placement of noninvasive ankle distractor.

lesions in and around the ankle joint. Camera and shaver portals are interchanged as needed to ensure adequate joint visualization and debridement.

Next, the articular surfaces are inspected to ensure any osteochondral lesions are identified and treated appropriately if present (**Fig. 6**). Adequate debridement of the lateral gutter must be performed to remove any impinging tissue and expose the anterior distal face of the fibula for accurate anchor placement (**Fig. 7**).[15,16] This debridement additionally provides a well-prepared surface for ligament adherence upon repair. The anterior face of the distal fibula should be partially denuded with the arthroscopic shaver to allow for anchor placement as well as capsule and ligamentous fibrosis after the completed repair.[15,16,37] Throughout the remainder of the procedure, the anteromedial portal is used as the viewing portal.

Through the anterolateral portal, the first suture anchor is drilled for and placed under arthroscopic visualization at the anterior face of the distal fibula. This insertion point should be just below the level of the distal tibial plafond.[15] Care is taken to not violate the medial or lateral cortex of the fibula. After the anchor is secured, the suture

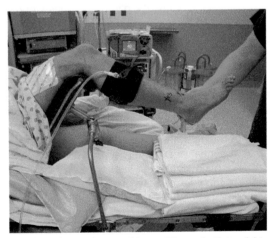

Fig. 5. Patient is placed in the supine position with an ipsilateral hip bump, and thigh holder.

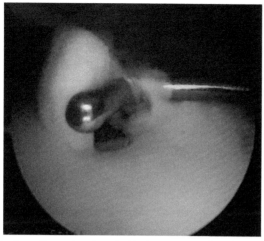

Fig. 6. Arthroscopic view of an osteochondral lesion that needs to be identified and treated appropriately prior to stabilization of the ankle.

ends then exit the anterolateral portal and are set aside. The second suture anchor is drilled for and placed approximately 1 cm distal to the previous anchor (**Fig. 8**). Spacing of the anchors is important so as to decrease risk for stress riser complication. After the anchor is secured, the suture ends then exit the anterolateral portal (**Fig. 9**).

For an inside-out technique, a sharp-tipped suture passer is then used to shuttle the 4 free suture ends through the lateral capsule, ligamentous structures (**Fig. 10**). The entry point of the suture passer should be confirmed via both external visualization of anatomic landmarks in addition to arthroscopic visualization upon entrance into the joint capsule. The suture ends attached to the inferior anchor will be used to reinforce the CFL distally. The suture attached to the superior suture will be used to reinforce the ATFL and incorporate the IER.

The first entry point of the suture passer is immediately superior to the peroneal tendons 5 mm distal to the fibula at the location of the insertion of the CFL on the

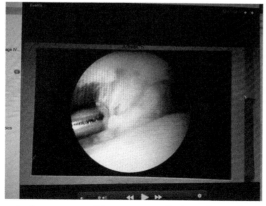

Fig. 7. An arthroscopic shaver us used to remove soft tissue from the anterior fibula.

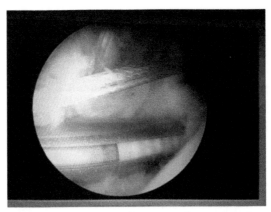

Fig. 8. Arthroscopic view of appropriate placement of suture anchors into the anterior fibula.

calcaneus and is placed with the foot in neutral dorsiflexion. The exit point is through the anterolateral portal. A wire loop is then used to pull one of the suture limbs from the inferior anchor out through the skin. The second entry point of the suture passer is approximately 5 mm anterior to the first suture pass and is again used to bring the other inferior-most suture end inferiorly out through or near the CFL. The third entry point of the suture passer is placed 1 cm dorsal to the peroneal tendons and 1.5 cm distal to the anterior surface of the fibula. The wire loop is now used to pull one of the suture limbs from the superior anchor out through the skin. The fourth entry point of the suture passer is approximately 1 cm dorsal to the third entry point along the arc of the IER.[15,16] Wire loop is used to now pull the second suture limb from the superior anchor out through the skin.

A skin incision approximately 3 to 4 mm wide is now made between the 2 sets of sutures oriented with Langer skin lines. A hemostat is used to gently separate the superficial subcutaneous soft tissue around the 4 sutures through this incision to prevent nerve and soft tissue impingement (**Fig. 11**). An arthroscopic probe is then used to pull all 4 suture limbs through this centrally placed incision (**Fig. 12**). The foot is then

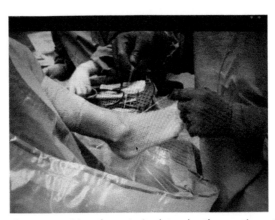

Fig. 9. Gross view of sutures exiting the anterior lateral arthroscopic portal.

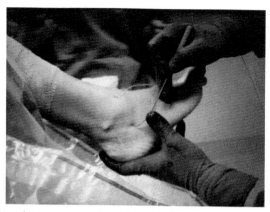

Fig. 10. A sharp tipped suture passer is used to shuttle the suture through the retinaculum and ankle capsule to reinforce the lateral ligaments.

held in dorsiflexion and eversion while the suture limbs are tied to their respective pair with either a surgeon's knot or arthroscopic slip knot. If puckering is present subcutaneous dissection is performed with a blunt hemostat through the distal skin incision to allow the skin to lie flat (**Fig. 13**). Free suture ends are now cut, and skin incisions are closed with nonabsorbable suture in a horizontal mattress fashion.

IMMEDIATE POSTOPERATIVE CARE

Operative extremity is placed in a below-knee posterior splint and kept nonweight bearing for 1 week. Sutures are removed at 10 to 14 days, and the patient is allowed to bathe at that time.

REHABILITATION AND RECOVERY

One week postoperatively, the patient is transitioned to full weight bearing in a full-length CAM walker with a night splint applied at night with the CAM

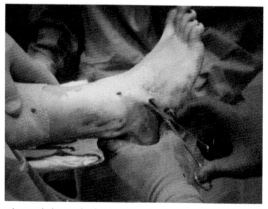

Fig. 11. A hemostat is used through the incision to free up the subcutaneous tissue, allowing for passage of suture and knot tying.

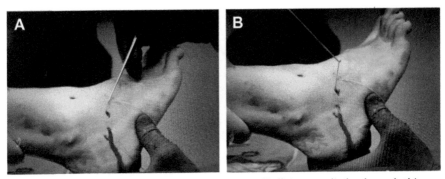

Fig. 12. An arthroscopic probe (*A*) is then used to pull all 4 suture limbs through this centrally placed incision (*B*).

walker removed. At this time, the patient is allowed to perform gentle dorsiflexion and plantarflexion range-of- motion exercises. Four to 6 weeks postoperatively, the patient is transitioned to full weight bearing in a sports brace. Six weeks postoperatively, nonballistic physical activity is allowed to tolerance, and 3 months postoperatively, running, jumping and other ballistic sport are allowed to tolerance.

CLINICAL RESULTS IN LITERATURE

Cottom and Rigby reported 1-year outcomes on 40 patients, showing an improvement in American Orthopedic Foot & Ankle Society (AOFAS) scores, from a mean 41.2 preoperatively to a postoperative mean of 95.4 with excellent stability and function noted.[16] Nery and colleagues[37] has the longest-term data on outcomes, reporting on a series of 38 patients with an average follow-up of 9.8 years, and their technique involved only 1 anchor in the fibula. The mean AOFAS at the final follow-up was 90, with 87% of patients returning to preinjury-level athletics. Acevedo and Mangon have quoted preliminary results of 73 patient who underwent the arthroscopic lateral ankle stabilization procedure, finding an improved Karlsson-Peterson score from a preoperative mean of 28.3 to a postoperative mean of 90.2.[15]

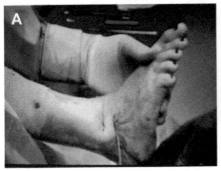
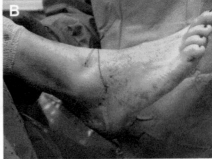

Fig. 13. (*A*) If puckering is present, subcutaneous dissection with a blunt hemostat through the distal skin incision allows the skin to lie flat. (*B*) Appearance after freeing subcutaneous tissue and incision closure.

SUMMARY

Ankle sprains are common injuries, and about 20% of patients will develop instability and may be candidates for surgical therapy.[3,4] Patient selection is also paramount to a good outcome. Patients with high body mass index and those with collagen deficiency disorders are relative contraindications to the arthroscopic ankle stabilization technique. Much of the procedure is percutaneous, and anatomic structures are not fully visualized. This necessitates a thorough knowledge of lateral ankle anatomic structures and safe zones. The arthroscopic lateral ankle stabilization technique has been shown to be safe and biomechanically equivalent to the open Bröstrom.[20] Choosing patients with virgin ligamentous laxity who have proven recalcitrant to appropriate conservative care for a minimum of 3 months after injury is indicated for success.[3,14,15,19,20,23,35,36]

REFERENCES

1. Waterman BR. The epidemiology of ankle sprains in the United States. J Bone Joint Surg Am 2010;92(13):2279.
2. Berlet GC, Anderson RB, Chron Davis W. Chronic lateral ankle instability. Foot Ankle Clin 1999;4:713–28.
3. Colville MR. Surgical treatment of the unstable ankle. J Am Acad Orthop Surg 1998;6(6):368–77.
4. Valderrabano V, Hintermann B, Horisberger M, et al. Ligamentous posttraumatic ankle osteoarthritis. Am J Sports Med 2006;34(4):612–20.
5. Freeman MA. Instability of the foot after injuries to the lateral ligament of the ankle. J Bone Joint Surg Br 1965;47(4):669–77.
6. Chan KW, Ding BC, Mroczek KJ. Acute and chronic lateral ankle instability in the athlete. Bull NYU Hosp Jt Dis 2011;69(1):17–26.
7. Harrington K. The role of the musculature in injuries to the medial collateral ligament. J Bone Joint Surg Am 1979;61(3):354–61.
8. Vogler HW, Bauer GR. Ankle fractures pathomechanics and treatment. In: Banks AS, Downey MS, Martin DE, et al, editors. Mcglamry's comprehensive textbook of foot and ankle surgery. 2nd edition. Philadelphia: Lippincott Williams & Wilkins; 2001.
9. DiGiovanni BF, Partal G, Baumhauer JF. Acute ankle injury and chronic lateral instability in the athlete. Clin Sports Med 2004;23(1):1–19.
10. Liu SH, Baker CL. Comparison of lateral ankle ligamentous reconstruction procedures. Am J Sports Med 1994;22(3):313–7.
11. Khawaji B, Soames R. The anterior talofibular ligament: a detailed morphological study. Foot (Edinb) 2015;25(3):141–7.
12. Burks RT, Morgan J. Anatomy of the lateral ankle ligaments. Am J Sports Med 1994;22:72–7.
13. Wainright WB, Spritzer CE, Lee JY, et al. The effect of modified Broström-Gould repair for lateral ankle instability on in vivo tibiotalar kinematics. Am J Sports Med 2013;40(9):2099–104.
14. Sammarco VJ. Complications of lateral ankle ligament reconstruction. Clin Orthop Relat Res 2001;391:123–32.
15. Acevedo JI, Mangone P. Ankle instability and arthroscopic lateral ligament repair. Foot Ankle Clin 2015;20(1):59–69.
16. Cottom JM, Rigby RB. The "all inside" arthroscopic Broström procedure: a prospective study of 40 consecutive patients. J Foot Ankle Surg 2013;52(5):568–74.

17. Peters JW, Trevino SG, Renstrom PA. Chronic lateral ankle instability. Foot Ankle 1991;12:182–91.
18. Acevedo JI, Ortiz C, Golano P, et al. ArthroBrostrom lateral ankle stabilization technique: an anatomic study. Am J Sports Med 2015;43(10):2564–71.
19. Chrisman OD, Snook GA. Reconstruction of lateral ligament tears of the ankle. An experimental study and clinical evaluation of seven patients treated by a new modification of the Elmslie procedure. J Bone Joint Surg Am 1969;51(5):904–12.
20. Komenda GA, Ferkel RD. Arthroscopic findings associated with the unstable ankle. Foot Ankle Int 1999;20(11):708–13.
21. Colville MR. Reconstruction of the lateral ankle ligaments. Instr Course Lect 1995; 44:341–8.
22. Bahr R, Pena F, Shine J, et al. Biomechanics of ankle reconstruction reconstruction technique. Am J Sports Med 1997;25(4):424–32.
23. Becker HP, Ebner S, Ebner D, et al. 12-year outcome after modified Watson-Jones tenodesis for ankle instability. Clin Orthop Relat Res 1999;358:194–204.
24. Brostrom L. Sprained ankles, VI: surgical treatment of "chronic" ligament ruptures. Acta Chir Scand 1966;243:551–65.
25. Gould N, Seligson D, Gassman J. Early and late repair of the lateral ligaments of the ankle. Foot Ankle 1980;1:84–9.
26. Sugimoto K. Chondral injuries of the ankle with recurrent lateral instability: an arthroscopic study. J Bone Joint Surg Am 2009;91(1):99.
27. Hamilton WG, Thompson FM, Snow SW. The modified Broström procedure for lateral ankle instability. Foot Ankle 1993;14(1):1–7.
28. Eyring DJ, Guthrie WD. A surgical approach to the problem of severe lateral instability at the ankle. Clin Orthop Relat Res 1986;206:185–91.
29. Taga I, Shino K, Inoue M, et al. Articular cartilage lesions in ankles with lateral ligament injury: an arthroscopic study. Am J Sports Med 1993;21:120–7.
30. Vega J, Golanó P, Pellegrino A, et al. All-inside arthroscopic lateral collateral ligament repair for ankle instability with a knotless suture anchor technique. Foot Ankle Int 2016;34(12):1701–9.
31. Drakos M, Behrens SB, Mulcahey MK, et al. Proximity of arthroscopic ankle stabilization procedures to surrounding structures: an anatomic study. Arthroscopy 2013;29(6):1089–94.
32. Giza E, Whitlow SR, Williams BT, et al. Biomechanical analysis of an arthroscopic broström ankle ligament repair and a suture anchor-augmented repair. Foot Ankle Int 2015;36:836–41.
33. Giza E, Shin EC, Wong SE, et al. Arthroscopic suture anchor repair of the lateral ligament ankle complex. Am J Sports Med 2013;41(11):2567–72.
34. Karlsson J, Bergsten T, Lansinger O, et al. Reconstruction of the lateral ligaments of the ankle for chronic lateral instability. J Bone Joint Surg Am 1988;70A:581–8.
35. Karlsson J, Eriksson B, Renstroml P. Subtalar instability of the foot. Scand J Med Sci Sports 1998;8:191–7.
36. Watson-Jones R. Fractures and joint injuries: recurrent forward dislocation of the ankle joint. 4th edition. Baltimore (MD): Williams & Wilkins; 1955.
37. Nery C, Raduan F, Del Buono A, et al. Arthroscopic-assisted Broström-Gould for chronic ankle instability: a long-term follow-up. Am J Sports Med 2011;39(11): 2381–8.

Small Joint Arthroscopy in the Foot

Christopher L. Reeves, DPM, FACFAS[a,b,]*, Amber M. Shane, DPM, FACFAS[b,c],
Trevor Payne, DPM[d], Zac Cavins, DPM[e]

KEYWORDS

- Arthroscopy • Small joint • Foot • First metatarsophalangeal joint
- Lesser metatarsal joints • Calcaneal cuboid joint • Talonavicular joint

KEY POINTS

- Arthroscopy has advanced in the foot and ankle realm, leading to new innovative techniques designed toward treatment of small joint abnormality.
- A range of abnormalities that are currently widespread for arthroscopic treatment in larger joints continues to be translated to congruent modalities in the small joints.
- Small joint arthroscopy offers relief from foot ailments with a noninvasive element afforded by arthroscopy.
- Early studies have found comparable results from arthroscopic soft tissue procedures as well as arthrodesis of the small joints when compared with the standard open approach.

INTRODUCTION

From its initial inception in the 1920s by Takagi[1] to investigate a knee infected with tuberculosis, and later refinement by Watanabe[2] with the advent of 2.2-mm and 1.7-mm fiber optic hardware, arthroscopy has made significant advancements toward a viable alternative for many open surgical interventions to correct pathologic processes in the body. As discussed by Oloff and colleagues,[3] the application of

Financial Disclosure: The authors have nothing to disclose as it relates to the content of this article.
Conflict of Interest: None reported.
[a] Orlando Foot and Ankle Clinic, 2111 Glenwood Drive, Suite 104, Winter Park, FL 32792, USA; [b] Surgical Residency Program, Department of Podiatric Surgery, Florida Hospital East Orlando, 7727 Lake Underhill Road, Orlando, FL 32828, USA; [c] Orlando Foot and Ankle Clinic, 250 North Alafaya Trail, Suite 115, Orlando, FL, USA; [d] Podiatric Medicine and Surgery Resident (PGY3), Residency Training Program, Florida Hospital East Orlando, 7727 Lake Underhill Road, Orlando, FL 32828, USA; [e] Podiatric Medicine and Surgery Resident (PGY1), Residency Training Program, Florida Hospital East Orlando, 7727 Lake Underhill Road, Orlando, FL 32828, USA
* Corresponding author. Orlando Foot and Ankle Clinic, 2111 Glenwood Drive, Suite 104, Winter Park, FL 32792.
E-mail address: creeves@orlandofootandankle.com

Clin Podiatr Med Surg 33 (2016) 565–580
http://dx.doi.org/10.1016/j.cpm.2016.06.005
0891-8422/16/$ – see front matter © 2016 Elsevier Inc. All rights reserved.

arthroscopy in the wrist has been detailed for some time, with a substantial deferment in correlative usage in the foot comparatively. Although used and embraced much later, arthroscopy in the foot and ankle has become a mainstay of treatment for the modern foot and ankle surgeon. Arthroscopy continues to break barriers with pioneers forging ahead, using new technique enhancements that have allowed the practice to progress with a focus on more advanced pathologic evaluation and treatment in the foot, including hallux abducto valgus, hallux limitus and rigidus, synovitis of the metatarsophalangeal joints, and arthritis throughout the Chopart joint. In short, arthroscopy is a minimally invasive alternative to open procedural techniques that can be wielded as a powerful tool. If used properly and safely, this modality can provide excellent outcomes for the patient with faster healing times and decreased risk of complications.

HISTORY

Wantanabe[2] in 1972 first described first metatarsophalangeal joint arthroscopy; since then, other authors have described treatment options that have provided patients with success. In 1996, Oloff and colleagues[3] described the results of a case series involving the diagnostic and therapeutic follow-up results of talonavicular and calcaneocuboid arthroscopy with good results. Details of safe access to the talonavicular joint were described by Hammond and colleagues[4] in 2011. They found that adequate debridement necessary for arthrodesis of this joint was feasible with a 2-portal technique.

INDICATIONS

Patient selection is always an important factor to take into consideration with arthroscopic intervention. Contraindications would include patients with poor arterial blood flow and cases where the procedure would be better performed as an open procedure. Also, there are specific abnormalities that can be addressed with arthroscopy. As arthroscopy of the foot and ankle becomes more commonplace, the type and complexity correctable abnormality by arthroscopy will broaden. Acceptance of arthroscopy in the ankle, subtalar joint, and first metatarsophalangeal joint is commonplace. However, the remaining lesser joints in the foot have scant literature on methodology and recommendations for surgical technique.[5] It is advised that a surgeon confident in their skills attempt an arthroscopic treatment for these less frequently attempted anatomic joints. A less experienced surgeon would be better suited to proceed with an open procedure, due to more exposure and practice in traditional training programs. In this case, an open procedure would theoretically have more risk of complications, but due to a lack of experience, would be more predictable in long-term results.

Indications for the first metatarsophalangeal joint arthroscopy include but are not limited to hallux rigidus, hallux valgus, arthrodesis, and joint synovectomy. There have been case reports listed for the treatment of arthrofibrosis, osteochondritis dissecans, and gout.[6-8] Similar indications are present for the lesser metatarsophalangeal joints and Chopart joint.[3,4]

PREOPERATIVE PLANNING

In order to optimize the potential outcomes of a procedure, many factors should be considered. An intimate anatomic knowledge of the foot, and particularly that around the joints involved with the arthroscopic portal sites, is of paramount importance. Neurovascular and tendinous tracts should be well understood and marked before any arthroscopic procedure. It is important to consider the size of the joint. For example, the first metatarsophalangeal joint is relatively small; therefore, a 1.9- or 2.3-mm arthroscope should be used in most cases.[6,9,10]

GENERAL ARTHROSCOPIC TECHNIQUE

Typically, anesthesia is initiated after intravenous sedation. Then, a pneumatic thigh or calf tourniquet is applied to provide an environment of a bloodless surgical field. The lower extremity is then scrubbed, prepped, and draped using normal aseptic technique. The surgeon should position himself and the patient to easily access the needed anatomic portals and manipulate the instrumentation. When positioning is finalized, the surgeon has the option to insufflate the joint with fluids. Insufflating the joint with fluids can be of benefit because distending the joint allows for easier penetration of blunt instrumentation to access the joint during portal placement. These authors recommend the use of lactated Ringer solution for insufflation into the joint because of its highly correlated physiologic properties to that of joint fluid.[11] In addition, the use of local anesthetics in the joint space is a common practice both with and without epinephrine. Previously described surgical techniques have highlighted its use preoperatively, intraoperatively, and postoperatively for pain reduction after surgery as well as additional hemostasis when epinephrine is used. However, literature has shown cell death of chondrocytes when exposed to local anesthetic mixtures for prolonged periods of time. Ropivacaine seems to be tolerated with the least side effects associated with chondrocyte mortality when compared with other options such as lidocaine and bupivacaine; therefore, anesthetic use should be tempered with the relative necessity of anticipated pain control needed after surgery.[11]

INSTRUMENTATION IN SMALL JOINT ARTHROSCOPY

Instrumentation for arthroscopy generally includes the arthroscope and associated light source with a monitor. In the small joints, gravity ingress of fluid is recommended due to the limited space of the joints encountered. The range in size of arthroscopes is from 1.5 mm in diameter to 2.7 mm in diameter when used in the small joints of the foot.[6,11] Typical motorized cutters, shavers, burrs, and abraders are used in the same fashion as other, larger joint spaces in a scaled-down version. In addition, a variety of hand instruments are available for arthroscopic manipulation and include graspers, probes, punches, rongeurs, and curettes. Radioablative wands are of valuable use for removing residual synovitis and excess tissue after the efficacy of traditional tools has been exhausted.[11]

FIRST METATARSOPHALANGEAL JOINT
Anatomy

The base of the proximal phalanx of the hallux is described as being ovoid in shape. The base of the proximal phalanx is wider medial to lateral than it is height dorsal to plantar. The surface is entirely concave medial to lateral and dorsal to plantar.[12] The head of the first metatarsal is rounded. The articular surface of the metatarsophalangeal joint is covered by hyaline cartilage, which also extends dorsally to aid in dorsiflexion and plantarly to the medial and lateral grooves, which allows for articulation with the sesamoids.[13]

The sesamoid bones serve as an attachment for the flexor hallucis brevis muscle and are attached to the metatarsal via the metatarsosesamoid ligaments and to the proximal phalanx of the hallux with the help of the phalangeal sesamoid ligaments.

The sesamoids are adhered to the plantar metatarsophalangeal ligament, which results in a firm attachment to the proximal phalanx. The tibial sesamoid provides an insertion point for the abductor hallucis, and the fibular sesamoid provides an insertion point for the adductor hallucis and the deep transverse metatarsal ligament.[13]

Innervation to the first metatarsophalangeal joint should be considered. The medial plantar hallucal nerve is just medial to the medial sesamoid. The common plantar digital nerve divides into lateral plantar hallucal nerve and can locate plantar and lateral-to-lateral sesamoid. The dorsal medial hallucal nerve, which is a branch of superficial peroneal nerve, runs medial to the extensor hallucis longus (EHL) tendon. The dorsal lateral hallucal nerve runs lateral to the EHL tendon and is considered a branch of the deep peroneal nerve.

Arthroscopic Anatomy

The hallux can be distracted either manually or via an external fixation device. The joint line can be determined by puckering of the skin. The puckering of the skin helps determine the place of both the dorsomedial and the dorsolateral portals. The EHL tendon is marked out throughout its course through the hallux (**Fig. 1**). A small incision is made longitudinally just medial to the EHL tendon. Blunt dissection is carried down to the level of the joint to avoid neurovascular injury. Once the joint is encountered, it is then insufflated with lactated Ringer solution. As insufflation continues, a blunt obturator is placed into the now created dorsomedial portal followed by portal, and then

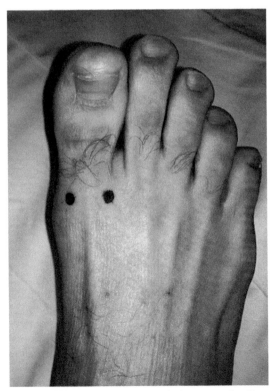

Fig. 1. Correct dorsomedial and dorsolateral portal placement for first metatarsal phalangeal joint access.

into the joint, followed by the arthroscope. As mentioned previously, the most common arthroscope for these small joints is a 2.3-mm or 1.9-mm arthroscope using 30° angulation. Following placement of the scope, an 18-gauge needle is inserted into the lateral portal site just lateral to the EHL tendon. Once placement is confirmed, a superficial skin incision is carried down, and blunt dissection into the capsule is again used to prevent neurovascular injury. A blunt obturator is then used to enter the dorsolateral portal to allow for better egress of fluid and placement of instruments.

The joint is then inspected, and a probe is used to evaluate the cartilage surface, evaluating for osteochondral lesions (OCDs), osteophytes, meniscal bodies, and inspection of the synovial recesses (**Fig. 2**). A 1.9- to 2.0-mm shaver or thermocoagulation may be required to remove hemorrhagic or hypertrophic synovitis within the joint (**Fig. 3**).

Siclari and Piras[14] described a 10-point intra-articular examination: the medial and lateral gutters, the medial and lateral corners of the metatarsal head, the central portion of the metatarsal head, the medial and lateral portion of the proximal phalanx, the central portion of the proximal phalanx, and the medial and lateral sesamoids.

Selected Procedures of the First Metatarsophalangeal Joint

Synovectomy
When addressing painful synovitis and pursuing synovectomy to ensure the most favorable outcome, it is recommended to place the shaver into both the dorsomedial and the dorsolateral portals and alternate removing the hypertrophic tissue that may be present. Consider use of thermal coagulation for hemorrhagic tissues. After the tissues are removed, confirm by investigating each aspect of the joint.

Hallux arthrosis
Similar to the removal of painful synovitis, when you have a patient with hallux rigidus, it is advised to place the shaver into both the dorsomedial and the dorsolateral portal

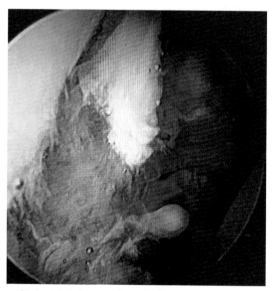

Fig. 2. Visualization of intrajoint abnormality of a first metatarsal phalangeal joint with meniscoid body and synovitis.

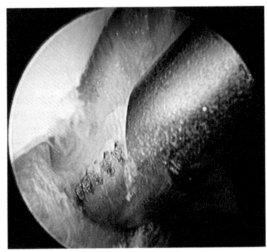

Fig. 3. Access with shaver for reduction of inflammatory tissue of a first metatarsal phalangeal joint.

and alternate removing the osteophytes that may be present along the first metatarsophalangeal joint. Occasionally, osteophytes will be encountered that are resistant to the shaver; in the scenario, one should consider the use of a burr for the bone spurs in addition to the shaver, if necessary. However, when using a burr, one must be cautious and avoid damaging healthy bone and cartilage that may be present within and around the joint.

Arthrodesis

The most important concept is to denude all of the cartilage on the head of the metatarsal and base of the proximal phalanx by using both a shaver and a burr. It is vital to the procedure to ensure that the subchondral surfaces are properly prepared. As mentioned previously, use of a burr within the joint must be performed with the strictest of attention so as not to remove too much. Once the joint is prepared, the joint is now able to accept 2 percutaneous screws to aid in the compression and fusion process.

LESSER METATARSOPHALANGEAL JOINTS

Pain associated with the lesser metatarsal phalangeal joints is a commonly encountered complaint. Patients present with a variety of issues not always easily isolated on physical examination. Arthroscopy is a good option to evaluate and treat typical abnormality associated with pain in these joints. The support structures of the joint, such as the collateral and proper ligaments, the plantar plate, associated tendons, and capsular integrity, can all be evaluated with arthroscopic inspection.[5,6,10] A clear understanding of the complete anatomic structure of the lesser metatarsophalangeal joint complex is crucial for successful implementation of corrective arthroscopic procedures.

Anatomy

The heads of the second, third, fourth, and fifth metatarsals have a convex shape and articulate with the concave proximal phalanx of the respective second, third, fourth, and fifth digits. The metatarsophalangeal joint capsule attaches in the groove adjacent to the articular surface both medially and laterally, and the proper collateral as well as the accessory collateral ligaments of that joint are attached to the metatarsal tubercles at the heads.[3] The floor of the lesser metatarsal phalangeal joints is made up of the plantar plate, which is an extension of the deep transverse intermetatarsal ligament. The plantar plate has a range of length from 16 mm to 23 mm with an average of 19 mm. The width of the plantar plate ranges from 8 mm to 13 mm with an average of 11 mm proximally and 9 mm distally.[10]

Arthroscopic Anatomy

A detailed summary of the arthroscopic anatomy was conducted by Nery and colleagues[10] in 2014 using cadaveric analysis. The report recommends entrance into the lesser metatarsophalangeal joints by 2 portals, specifically, dorsomedial and dorsolateral (**Fig. 4**). Insufflation of the joint with lactated Ringer solution is recommended before insertion of the obturator followed by the arthroscopy camera and specific wand types. The portal placement should then be conducted using a percutaneous incision just distal to the joint line. Blunt dissection into the joint is followed by integration of the inserted 18-gauge needle with a pump system to maintain distraction of the joint. Recommended arthroscope size is 2.7 or 1.9 mm.[6]

  Positioning for this procedure should be in the normal fashion, with the addition of finger traps; the digits with the foot should be raised off of the bed for gravity-assisted distraction. During video observation, the first structure to be visualized is the plantar plate, which should have a color constant with the surrounding cartilage (**Fig. 5**). Any deviation from normal is concerning for underlying abnormality. Direct medial and lateral insertion of the plantar plate into the proximal phalanx is easily visualized. A probe should assess the central insertional region because this portion of the plantar

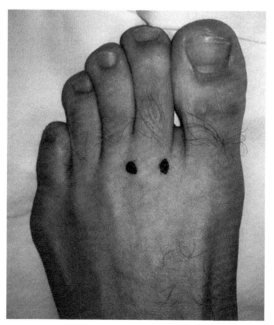

Fig. 4. Proper dorsomedial and dorsolateral placement of portals for arthroscopic entry.

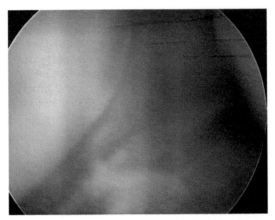

Fig. 5. Visual inspection of a lesser (second) metatarsal phalangeal joint.

plate passes in a recess and can give the false impression of an underlying tear (**Fig. 6**). Next, visualization of the medial and lateral accessory collateral ligaments is conducted by probing along the inferior border of the ligament's interface with the plantar plate. The ligaments have an inverted fan shape and terminate in the metatarsal tubercle bilaterally. From here, the surgeon should appreciate the proper collateral ligaments originating from the same site and incorporating as a thickened band that progresses externally and attaches to the base of the proximal phalanx.[10]

Selected Procedures of the Lesser Metatarsophalangeal Joints

Painful synovitis of the metatarsophalangeal joints is a common abnormality. Once conservative options have failed to alleviate symptoms, the decision point for a more invasive procedure must be initiated. Traditionally, an open procedure to visualize and remove the offending inflammatory tissue is used. An arthroscopic alternative is a viable way to address the abnormality without the invasive risk and possible side effects of an open modality.

Arthroscopic treatment begins by locating the joint space via penetration with 25-gauge guide needle into the previously described dorsomedial and dorsolateral

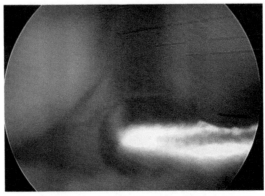

Fig. 6. Introduction of probe to manipulate tissue for better visualization of the normal joint anatomy.

positions on either side of the long extensor tendon. Once visualization of the joint space is achieved with insertion of the scope, a full inspection of the joint is advised with visualization of the cartilaginous, ligament, and capsular integrity. Switching between portal sites and rotation of the angular arthroscope can facilitate full visualization of the joint space. The medial and lateral gutters can be best visualized with the use of a 1.5-mm arthroscope, and reduction of inflammatory tissue can be conducted with use of a minishaver (**Fig. 7**). Special attention to the proximal aspect of the gutters (lateral, medial, and plantar) is essential because this area contains the highest degree and density of synovitis. Residual inflammatory tissue can be further reduced by use of a radioablative wand; however, care should be taken to avoid direct contact with the cartilaginous surface of the metatarsal head and corresponding phalanx base.[6]

Freiberg disease is a debilitating abnormality that can lead to significant reduction in quality of life due to pain and limitation of functional ability. Consensus of the cause of Freiberg disease is not fully agreed on, and several factors have been attributed to the disease, including mechanical forces, traumatic fracture of the subchondral bony architecture, microtrauma, and aseptic necrosis. It is generally accepted, however, that the disease stems from an osteochondrosis of the growing epiphysis. Several treatment options have been described from conservative to surgical.[6,8,15] Traditionally, surgical treatment was performed in an open fashion to treat the patient nonresponsive to conservative care. Recently, an arthroscopic treatment method has been detailed by Lui and Yuen.[6] Their team used the concept of an open interpositional arthroplasty and applied that technique to an arthroscopic correlative procedure.

The procedure is detailed by placing the appropriate portals in the dorsomedial and dorsolateral position. Debridement of any damaged cartilage is conducted, followed by a thorough synovectomy. An interpositional arthroplasty is then performed using the extensor digitorum brevis. The tendon is transected proximally to the joint with an auxiliary stab incision. The tendon is then gathered into the joint space and pulled externally through the dorsolateral portal and tethered into a ball structure with absorbable suture. Subsequently, the ball is reinserted into the joint space with an

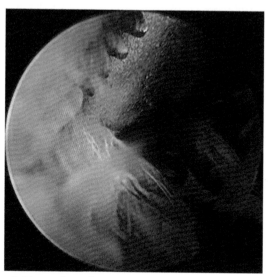

Fig. 7. Access with minishaver for reduction of synovitic tissue in a lesser metatarsal phalangeal joint.

eyed needle, which is arthroscopically guided through the plantar plate and out of the bottom of the foot. The suture is tied off plantarly, suspending the interpositional tissue and restoring joint space.[6]

CHOPART JOINT

The Chopart joint or "transverse tarsus joint" comprises the talonavicular and calcaneocuboid joints. The joint was championed as a viable amputation location by François Chopart in the eighteenth century. These joints have important balancing properties that allow translation of movement from the lower leg and rearfoot to the remainder of the foot complex. In addition, the Chopart joint is responsible for allowing the maintenance of medial and lateral columns during motion. The talocalcaneal joint has the most available motion of the 2 joints, and with its additional articulation to the calcaneus (coxa pedis), allows for most eversion and inversion of the midfoot and forefoot. As opposed to the 3-joint medial column complex, the lateral column is made up of just 2 joints; however, the calcaneocuboid joint allows for concurrent flexibility and stabilization of the midfoot/rearfoot interface during ambulation, which in unison act to allow pivoting along the longitudinal axis of the foot and has been described as a screwlike motion.[15,16] It has been reported that possible indications for arthroscopy in these joints include management of osteochondritis dissecans, loose body removal, inflammatory and noninflammatory synovitis, osteophyte reduction, synovial impingement, infection, and biopsy and aid in visual diagnosis.[3]

TALONAVICULAR JOINT
Anatomy

The head of the talus articulates by an interphase in the shape of a socket formed by the posterior surface of the navicular, the anterior and middle talar articular facets of the calcaneus, and the plantar calcaneonavicular ligament. In addition to the ligaments incorporated into the capsule, the talocalcaneonavicular joint is reinforced by the anterior-most fibers of the deltoid ligament and by the calcaneonavicular slip of the bifurcate ligament. The head of the talus is convex in all directions, but it is not a segment of a sphere.[13] The dorsalis pedis artery and the deep branch of the peroneal nerve are in close approximation to the dorsal aspect of the joint, while the saphenous vein and nerve cross at a more dorsal medial attitude. The tibialis anterior, EHL, and extensor digitorum longus cross the joint dorsally, whereas the posterior tibial tendon crosses plantar medially. The calcaneocuboid joint is colinear with the lateral joint line and moves in conjunction with the talonavicular joint. The talonavicular joint is a key joint in motion of the hindfoot second only to the ankle joint. The talonavicular joint if fused will prevent almost all motion at the calcaneocuboid and subtalar joints.[15,16]

Arthroscopic Anatomy

Typical arthroscopic portals are placed in a medial, dorsomedial, and dorsolateral position (**Fig. 8**). The portal placements are confirmed with a 25-gauge needle before dissection and should penetrate the joint space. The medial portal position is accessed immediately dorsal to the posterior tibial tendon insertion at the joint line. The dorsolateral portal is placed at the junction of the talonavicular and calcaneocuboid joints. The medial portal should be placed at a midpoint between the dorsolateral and dorsomedial portals. Of the 3 portals, the dorsomedial has the highest likelihood of proximity to nerve structures.[6] Superficial stab incisions should be made in a longitudinal fashion and dissected bluntly to the joint space to avoid iatrogenic transection of vital structures. Between access to all 3 portals and the use of eversion

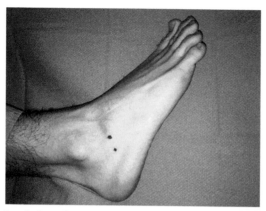

Fig. 8. Three-portal technique for adequate visualization of the talonavicular joint.

intraoperatively, the great majority of the joint can be visualized, inspected, and addressed as indicated.

Selected Procedures of Chopart Joint

There have been several reports on cadaveric specimens detailing the viability of an arthrodesis procedure of the talonavicular joint.[6,9,10] Traditionally done in an open fashion, it is a vital component of the triple or double arthrodesis procedure by eliminating most of the hindfoot range of motion. It is often indicated in patients suffering from arthritic pain resulting from degenerative, traumatic, rheumatologic, and deformity-driven factors such as untreated pediatric flatfoot. Patients with conditions requiring joint arthrodesis are candidates for arthroscopic treatment. Advantages to this modality include complete visualization of the talonavicular joint because it is the most common site of nonunion due to difficulty in reaching the plantar and lateral aspect of the talar joint with traditional open dissection. In contrast, talonavicular arthrodesis via arthroscopy has the potential advantage of better intra-articular visualization, and more complete cartilage debridement and preservation of subchondral bone.[9]

Systematic debridement of the visualized cartilaginous surface should be done in a sweeping fashion from medial to lateral along the navicular with corresponding use of the dorsolateral, dorsomedial, and medial portals. The same stepwise process should be used to visualized and subsequently reduce the cartilage of the talar head (**Fig. 9**), and this is best achieved with the use of a 3-mm shaver (**Fig. 10**). Hammond and colleagues[4] reported an average articular surface debridement area of 98.6% of the navicular and 83.2% to the talus. Once all of the cartilage has been removed, the surgeon should replace the shaver with a burr and resect the remaining subchondral plate. The portals can be used for insertion of any advanced allograft or bone-stimulating products while still under visualization. At this point, a variety of percutaneous screw fixation options are available to hold stability and compression across the joint space.

Addressing OCDs with arthroscopy in the talonavicular joint has been shown to be a viable alternative to its traditionally open counterpart.[3,4,17,18] Although rare, OCD lesions of the talonavicular joint are debilitating and usually require an open approach with extensive soft tissue dissection. Microfracture treatment with arthroscopy has

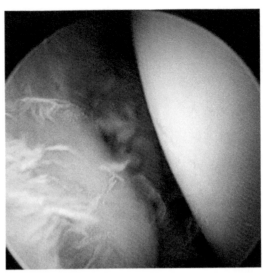

Fig. 9. Visualization of the talonavicular joint with prominent talar head and synovitic inflammatory tissue.

been widely reported and used in the ankle. The same approach can be taken when addressing an OCD lesion of the talonavicular joint.

The procedure begins with arthroscopic visualization of the joint as described above along with confirmation and analysis of the OCD lesion itself. Visualization can be further improved by use of a Hintermann distraction device. Kirschner wires typically measuring 0.062 inches are inserted into the neck of the talus and body of the navicular in the dorsomedial position with care taken to avoid penetration into or near the cartilaginous structures. Intraoperative fluoroscopy can be useful as a visual guide

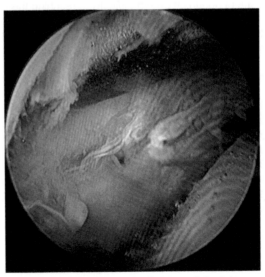

Fig. 10. Utilization of the shaver for better visualization of the joint space via reduction of inflammatory tissue in the talonavicular joint.

during pin insertion. Debridement of an OCD lesion is best conducted with a curette and shaver. Following this, microfracture with an awl through the subchondral bone will allow for bleeding and eventual infiltration of fibrocartilage into the joint.[17]

CALCANEOCUBOID JOINT

As compared with other, more well-investigated arthroscopic techniques of the foot, such as the subtalar joint and first metatarsophalangeal joints, there is scarce literature available detailing the use of arthroscopy in the calcaneocuboid joint. Perhaps this is due to the infrequency of isolated abnormality, the relative difficulty in accessing the joint, and the limited number of surgeons using this modality in favor of more well-studied and predictable open procedures.

Anatomy

The calcaneocuboid joint is formed by the posterior surface of the cuboid and the anterior surface of the calcaneus. It plays a role in triplanar motion between the talo-navicular and subtalar joints. It is surrounded by a host of soft tissue structures. On the plantar aspect of the foot it is surrounded by the long and short plantar ligaments and peroneus longus tendon. Dorsal support is achieved by the combined bifurcate and calcaneocuboid ligaments. The calcaneocuboid joint is described as a saddle joint.[13] The sural nerve lies just lateral to the joint, and the intermediate superficial branch of the peroneal nerve branches lie slightly dorsal as well as the extensor digitorum brevis. The joint has a tight lateral and plantar capsule because it is instrumental in supporting the arch of the foot and maintaining the integrity of the lateral column. The joint has a complex "S"-shaped surface, allowing some medial to lateral as well as dorsiflexion and plantarflexion translation motion.

Arthroscopic Anatomy

There are 2 interchangeable portal placements that are designated as superior and inferior. The superior portal is best approached at the level of the anterior process of the calcaneus with the inferior portal being 2 to 3 cm below that of the superior portal in line with the joint and superior to the peroneus brevis tendon (**Fig. 11**). Lui and colleagues[6] consider the calcaneocuboid portal placement "the most important portal of midtarsal arthroscopy because the medial aspect of the CC joint, the lateral and plantar aspects of the TN joint, the anterior subtalar joint, and the junction between

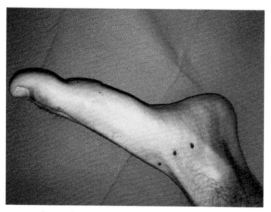

Fig. 11. Portal placement for arthroscopic access to the calcaneocuboid joint.

the talus, calcaneus, navicular, and cuboid can be reached through this portal." Again, intraoperative fluoroscopy can be useful in triangulating the placement of 25-gauge needles. Distention of the joint can be conducted with an 18-gauge needle and lactated Ringer solution. Superficial skin incisions are recommended in the longitudinal plane with use of blunt dissection through the joint capsule with special attention to avoid the sural and intermediate dorsal cutaneous nerves. Placement of a 2.3-mm 30° scope has been reported (**Fig. 12**). Utilization of shavers, probes, burrs, radioablative tools, and cutters can be conducted interchangeably[6] (**Fig. 13**).

Selected Procedures of the Calcaneocuboid Joint

Isolation of abnormality to the calcaneocuboid joint can be achieved by a diagnostic anesthetic injection. Once confirmed, the role of arthroscopy can help to further diagnose the cause of the patient complaints. Through the use of both portals, evaluation of joint spaces, degrees of synovitis, inspection for loose bodies, and visualization of osteochondral defects can be achieved. OCD lesions can be addressed with microfracture with the same general protocol used in the talonavicular and other joints. Primary arthrodesis, to the best of the authors' knowledge, has not been reported in the literature. However, Lui and colleagues[9] published a case report in 2013 highlighting the treatment of a calcaneocuboid distraction arthrodesis nonunion using arthroscopy. Loosening and removal of the fibrotic nonunion was conducted with a probe and shaver, whereas the bony interface was freshened with a curette, arthroscopic burr, and arthroscopic awl. The 2 portals were used as entry points for autologous graft. Twelve weeks postoperatively, the site was fused without difficulty or limitation of function.

POSTOPERATIVE COURSE

The arthroscopic portals are closed using 4-0 nylon suture in a horizontal mattress suture pattern. A nonadherent petrolatum gauze dressing and 4 × 4 gauze pads are placed, and the ankle is immobilized in a well-padded splint in neutral dorsiflexion. The sutures and splint are removed in 7 days.[19] The postoperative course is determined by the type of the procedure and the general abilities of the patient. If the patient

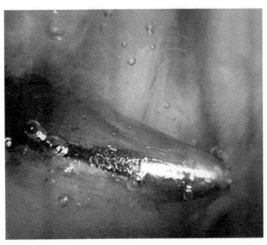

Fig. 12. Visualization of the calcaneocuboid joint with associated inflammatory tissue.

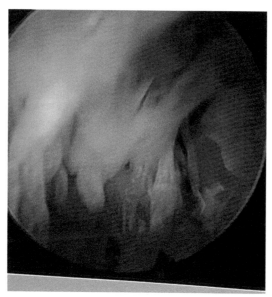

Fig. 13. Enhanced visualization of the calcaneocuboid joint with use of an arthroscopic probe.

has undergone a simple arthroscopic synovectomy or hallux rigidus procedure, the patient may typically weight-bear as tolerated while wearing a postoperative shoe. However, if the patient had undergone an arthrodesis, it would be realistic to consider restricting weight-bearing for several weeks until the bone has a chance show signs of cross-bridging.

COMPLICATIONS

Complications from arthroscopy are contingent on many factors, such as the relative experience of the surgeon, the joint space addressed, and the degree of involvement of the procedure required, and can include infection, nerve or vascular injury from improper placement of portals, articular cartilage damage, and compartment ischemia. Following sterile technique will help in reducing the chance for infection, and knowledge of specific joint anatomy can help reduce unnecessary soft tissue and nerve damage. As mentioned in numerous sections above, careful dissection and attention especially when using the power burr or radioablative tool can decrease the chance of cartilage damage. Careful monitoring of the patient is necessary during the immediate postoperative course and is easily done so due to its minimally invasive nature.[20]

SUMMARY

Arthroscopic management of the lesser joints of the foot is a specialized technique and should not be performed by the occasional arthroscopist. Like any surgical procedure, it should be performed when the appropriate indications are present and addressed with appropriate technique. This procedure has a favorable outcome with minimal complications. The benefits are truly magnified when one considers that these procedures result in a shortened hospitalization time, less pain as a result of the minimal surgical dissection and soft tissue stripping, and faster rehabilitation times. As more research becomes available, these aforementioned procedures could become mainstays in treatment of the discussed deformities.

REFERENCES

1. Takagi K. Practical experiences using Takagi's arthroscope. J Jpn Orthop Ass 1933;8:132.
2. Watanabe MB. History of arthroscopic surgery [Chapter 2]. Philadelphia: Lippincott; 1984.
3. Oloff L, Schulhofer SD, Fanton G, Fanton G. Arthroscopy of the calcaneocuboid and talonavicular joints. J Foot Ankle Surg 1996;35(2):101–8.
4. Hammond AW, Phisitkul P, Femino J, et al. Arthroscopic debridement of the talonavicular joint using dorsomedial and dorsolateral portals: a cadaveric study of safety and access. Arthroscopy 2011;27(2):228–34.
5. Derner R, Naldo J. Small joint arthroscopy of the foot. Clin Podiatr Med Surg 2011;28(3):551–60.
6. Lui TH, Yuen CP. Small joint arthroscopy in foot and ankle. Foot Ankle Clin 2015; 20(1):123–38.
7. Wood DA, Christensen JC, Schuberth JM. The use of arthroscopy in acute foot and ankle trauma: a review. Foot Ankle Spec 2014;7(6):495–506.
8. Hayashi K, Ochi M, Uchio Y, et al. A new surgical technique for treating bilateral Freiberg disease. Arthroscopy 2002;18(6):660–4.
9. Lui TH, Chan LK. Safety and efficacy of talonavicular arthroscopy in arthroscopic triple arthrodesis. A cadaveric study. Knee Surg Sports Traumatol Arthrosc 2010; 18(5):607–11.
10. Nery C, Coughlin MJ, Baumfeld D, et al. Lesser metatarsal phalangeal joint arthroscopy: anatomic description and comparative dissection. Arthroscopy 2014;30(8):971–9.
11. Jennings MM, Bark SE. Practical aspects of foot and ankle arthroscopy. Clin Podiatr Med Surg 2011;28(3):441–52.
12. Carreira DS. Arthroscopy of the hallux. Foot Ankle Clin 2009;14:105–14.
13. Hirsch BE. Anatomy of the lower extremity. Philadelphia: Elsevier; 2005.
14. Siclari A, Piras M. Hallux metatarsophalangeal arthroscopy: indications and techniques. Foot Ankle Clin 2015;20:109–22.
15. Maresca G, Adriani E, Falez F, et al. Arthroscopic treatment of bilateral Freiberg's infraction. Arthroscopy 1996;12(1):103–8.
16. Seringe R, Wicart P, French Society of Pediatric Orthopaedics. The talonavicular and subtalar joints: the "calcaneopedal unit" concept. Orthop Traumatol Surg Res 2013;99(Suppl 6):S345–55.
17. Schneiders W, Rammelt S. Joint-sparing corrections of malunited Chopart joint injuries. Foot Ankle Clin 2016;21(1):147–60.
18. Ross KA, Seaworth CM, Smyth NA. Talonavicular arthroscopy for osteochondral lesions: technique and case series. Foot Ankle Int 2014;35(9):909–15.
19. Ferkel RD, Dierckman BD, Phisitkul P. Arthroscopy of the foot and ankle. Mann's Surgery of the Foot and Ankle. Elsevier; 2014. p. 1723–827.
20. Lamy C, Stienstra J. Complications in ankle arthroscopy. Arthroscopy 1994;11(3): 523–39.

Arthroscopic Ankle Arthrodesis

Byron Hutchinson, DPM

KEYWORDS

• Arthrodesis • Ankle • Arthroscopy • Fusion • Arthritis • Foot and ankle

KEY POINTS

- Arthroscopic ankle arthrodesis is a cost-effective option for many patients with posttraumatic arthritis of the ankle joint.
- Rehabilitation is generally quicker than conventional open techniques, and rates of fusion are comparable or better than traditional open techniques.
- Unless the arthroscopic surgeon has considerable experience, the best results are seen in patients with very little deformity in the ankle joint.

Ankle arthrodesis is arguably the best option in young and active patients affected by end-stage ankle arthritis.[1–3] There have been numerous open techniques described, and many of these techniques are used routinely by foot and ankle surgeons because of a familiarity with a particular technique or because of certain advantages a certain technique might provide in more complex deformities.[4] Total ankle replacement has gained popularity because of technological advancements in design and techniques, but is generally reserved for older, less active patients.[5–8]

Since its description in 1983, arthroscopic ankle fusion has gained popularity in selected patients.[9] Arthroscopic ankle arthrodesis has demonstrated faster union rates, decreased complications, reduced postoperative pain, and shorter hospital stays.[1,2,9–12] Advancements in techniques and instrumentation have allowed this procedure to gain popularity with foot and ankle surgeons that have considerable arthroscopic training and experience.

ADVANTAGES OF ARTHROSCOPIC ANKLE ARTHRODESIS
Indications and Contraindications

Arthroscopic ankle arthrodesis is primarily indicated in patients with end-stage ankle arthritis. In 2005, Saltzman and colleagues[13] reviewed 693 patients with end-stage ankle arthritis and found that 79% of these patients suffered from posttraumatic

Highline Clinic, 16323 Sylvester Road Southwest G-10, Seattle, WA 98166, USA
E-mail address: byronhutchinson@chifranciscan.org

Clin Podiatr Med Surg 33 (2016) 581–589
http://dx.doi.org/10.1016/j.cpm.2016.06.006
0891-8422/16/$ – see front matter © 2016 Elsevier Inc. All rights reserved.

podiatric.theclinics.com

arthritis; 12% were associated with rheumatoid disease, and only 7% suffered from primary osteoarthritis. This study did not focus on the amount of deformity or bone loss within the various categories of end-stage ankle arthritis.

In the author's opinion, despite all the advantages seen with arthroscopic ankle arthrodesis, this technique should be considered only as an in situ fusion in most situations (**Fig. 1**). Certainly, there are several reports focused on extending arthroscopic ankle arthrodesis to correcting significant angular deformity and/or bone loss.[14,15] With the appropriate surgical experience, positive outcomes may be realized with significant angular deformity and/or bone loss, but this must be weighed against the advantages of other more traditional open techniques (**Fig. 2**).

One of the best advantages of arthroscopic ankle arthrodesis is in those situations wherein the skin envelope is poor or when there is excessive scarring (**Fig. 3**). The scarring can be from previous surgeries or from skin grafting. Arthroscopic ankle arthrodesis preserves blood supply by its very nature, and this is advantageous to a skin envelope, which may already be compromised. It is much easier to avoid areas of scar using small stab incisions versus traditional skin incisions in all open techniques. This technique can be beneficial in the elderly population because of the small incisions, faster union rates, and postoperative rehabilitation as discussed later in this article.

The technique is generally contraindicated in the presence of infection, excessive bone loss such as avascular necrosis of the talus, or in the presence of significant rigid intrinsic deformity of the ankle joint.

PREOPERATIVE EVALUATION

The most important consideration in the evaluation for an arthroscopic ankle arthrodesis is the status of all adjacent joints.[16,17] These joints will be required to compensate for the lack of motion at the ankle and should be free of degenerative changes. If there are deformities in the tibia, then it is important to address them at the time of surgery or before performing the arthroscopic ankle arthrodesis. Another consideration is

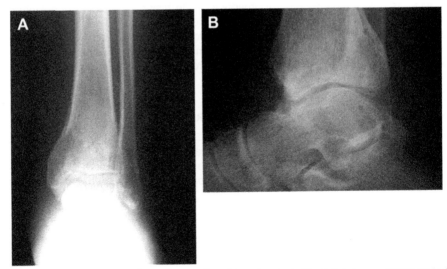

Fig. 1. An ideal ankle joint for arthroscopic ankle arthrodesis. The joint demonstrates typical arthritic changes with little or no deformity (*A, B*).

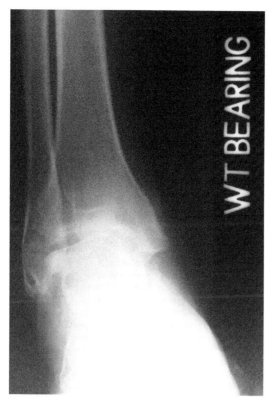

Fig. 2. Anteroposterior radiograph of the ankle shows the typical deformity in the ankle that the author finds is much more difficult to do arthroscopically unless the arthroscopic surgeon has significant experience.

whether there is any deformity or arthritis in the knee that needs to be addressed. In many circumstances, a total knee replacement and/or correction should be done before the arthroscopic ankle arthrodesis. The presence of tarsal mobility is paramount, and any fixed frontal or sagittal plane deformity in the forefoot will lead to a less than optimal result and should be considered[3] (**Fig. 4**).

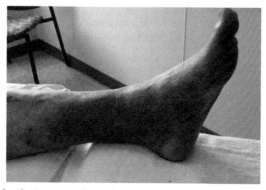

Fig. 3. The type of soft tissue envelope that is at risk with open arthrodesis techniques.

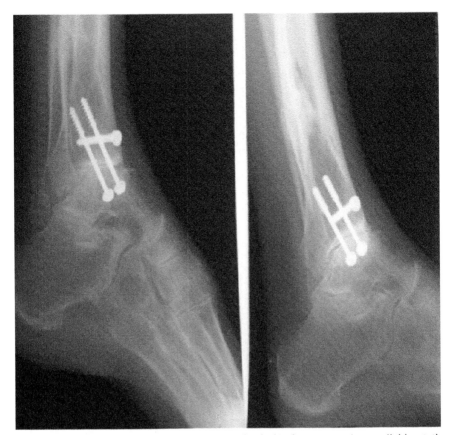

Fig. 4. These lateral radiographs demonstrate the lack of compensation available at the midfoot due to arthritis and deformity within these joints and can impact the success of any ankle fusion.

DIAGNOSTIC STUDIES

Plain radiographs are essential in the evaluation of the ankle. Weight-bearing antero-posterior, lateral, and mortise views of both ankles are required. If there is concern about the status of the joints of the midfoot, then additional radiographs of the foot should be obtained. If significant diaphyseal deformity is present, then in addition to ankle radiographs, long leg films and/or scanograms should be considered. The rear-foot alignment views will help to evaluate the ankle joint and identify any calcaneal to tibial deformities (**Fig. 5**).

Computed tomography (CT) and MRI scans are useful when evaluating bone defects or the soft tissue envelope. The author has also found Spect-CT (single photon emission computed tomography) to be extremely useful in those patients that may have concomitant degenerative changes in the subtalar and/or midtarsal joint (**Fig. 6**).

SURGICAL TECHNIQUE

The patient is placed supine under general or spinal anesthesia. Preoperative intravenous antibiotic prophylaxis is recommended. The author prefers to use a thigh tourniquet set at 300 to 350 mm Hg. An ipsilateral bump is placed under the hip to allow for

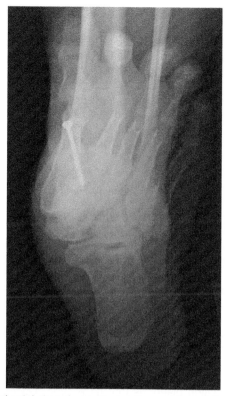

Fig. 5. A long calcaneal axial view demonstrates the position of the calcaneus in relationship to the long axis of the tibia.

the ankle to be in the most optimal position for performing the arthroscopic ankle arthrodesis. The author rarely uses distraction of the ankle, but in some circumstances, noninvasive distraction can be helpful. Invasive distraction is rarely used anymore because of the potential for stress fractures and/or nerve injury. Insufflation of the ankle joint can be obtained with a gravity bag of normal saline or lactated Ringer

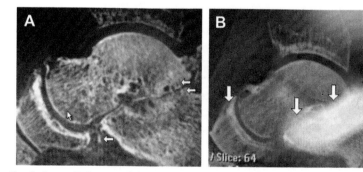

Fig. 6. Spect-CT image of the subtalar joint indicating that the area of uptake corresponds to the arthritic subtalar joint (*A*). Note the lack of uptake in some of the talonavicular joint (*B*). The arrows indicate arthritic changes.

solution. Commercially available arthroscopy bumps can also be used, but, in the author's opinion, are not necessary.

The ankle joint is insufflated with 30 to 50 mL of lactated Ringer or saline into the anterior ankle pouch. Arthroscopy is performed through 2 anterior portals: one medial and one lateral. The arthroscopic surgeon must be aware of the intermediate dorsal cutaneous nerve and the saphenous vein so as not to damage these structures. The 4.0-mm, 30° arthroscope is used in the vast majority of cases. A 70° scope can be used to visualize the posterior aspect of the joint and the gutters.

Initially, the anterior ankle pouch is debrided with a 3.5 full-radius resector to allow visualization of the joint surfaces. Anterior osteophytes may need to be removed, and this can be accomplished with a burr or with a small osteotome through one of the portals. A large burr and/or curettes are used to remove the remaining cartilage on the adjacent joint surfaces, usually starting on the talus. A systematic removal of the cartilage can now be done, by "mowing the lawn" so as not to leave islands of cartilage (**Fig. 7**). One will notice that the access to the joint improves once this cartilage is removed, and better access of the posterior aspect of the joint can now be obtained. Abrasion of the subchondral bone plate below the tidemark will allow for intra-articular bleeding to promote fusion. The talofibular aspect of the joint can also be removed to help in positioning of the talus during fixation.[3] The tourniquet can be released at this point to assess the bleeding from the tibial and talar surfaces.

Alignment and fixation of the joint can now be accomplished. Position of fusion is the same in arthroscopic ankle arthrodesis as any other technique: neutral position in the sagittal plane with the talus rocked posterior and the lateral talar process parallel to the long axis of the tibia. In the frontal plane there should be about 0° to 5° of valgus and 10° external rotation of the talus in the mortise. This alignment is determined with the tibial tuberosity being parallel to the second metatarsal phalangeal joint.

There are several fixation platforms that have been described.[3,9,11,12] The most important aspects of fixation are to eliminate the force of the gastrosoleus complex by having adequate anterior fixation and to spread the remaining fixation out over the entire joint surface. Too often the fixation intersects in the center of the joint so there is a rotational moment around the fixation, causing too much micromotion. The author prefers a percutaneous 3-screw approach with the first screw delivered

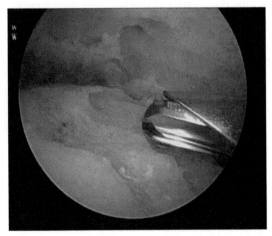

Fig. 7. The rotating burr removing cartilage and subchondral bone to promote fusion. This is being done from lateral to medial in rows similar to "mowing the lawn."

behind the fibula from posterolateral to anteromedial toward the talar neck. This so-called homerun screw can be difficult to place; sometimes the author will abandon this screw in favor of a 2-screw construct. The second screw is delivered from the medial malleolus to the lateral process of the talus, incorporating the medial bend of the joint. The final screw is placed anterolateral to posterior into the talus, providing some stability to the anterior joint line to counterbalance the pull of the gastrosoleus complex. Fluoroscopic visualization is necessary to achieve proper fixation. Proper fixation is of paramount importance in the author's opinion to prevent nonunion. The author prefers the use of the C-arm to accomplish proper fixation.

POSTOPERATIVE COURSE

The postoperative course can vary tremendously and is region and surgeon driven. The author uses a modified Jones compression splint for 5 to 7 days of non-weight-bearing until the first dressing change in the office when this is replaced with a removable cast boot and non-weight-bearing for another 5 weeks. Transition to weight-bearing in the cast boot occurs over the next 4 to 6 weeks, increasing weight-bearing to tolerance. Serial radiographs are taken at 2, 6, and 12 weeks. Physical therapy is used if necessary, and transition to activities of daily living as well as recreational activities occurs over the next 6 to 12 months.

DISCUSSION

In the past 2 decades, arthroscopic ankle fusion has gained popularity as an index procedure because of several advantages over traditional open techniques.

The fact that the procedure is "minimally invasive" lends itself to much better control of postoperative pain. Zvijac and colleagues[10] reported on 21 patients with a mean age of 52.7 years who underwent arthroscopic ankle fusion. This retrospective study had a follow-up time of 34 months, and fusion occurred in 20 of 21 patients. With regard to pain, 9 patients had no pain, and 11 had only mild pain during and after the procedure.

Myerson and Quil[2] compared arthroscopic ankle arthrodesis to an open method and demonstrated that there was less morbidity and a faster return to a normal life after arthroscopic ankle arthrodesis. In 2010, Peterson and colleagues[11] showed reduced cost compared with open ankle arthrodesis. There was a statistically significant difference between the cost of an arthroscopic ankle fusion done as an outpatient or at most a 1-day stay versus an open technique that typically requires 2 to 3 days in the hospital.

One of the main parameters in evaluating the efficacy of ankle arthrodesis is the rate of fusion. Fusion rates in ankle arthrodesis can be assessed by several clinical parameters. The presence of a clinically stable ankle, which is painless with weight-bearing, is a good indicator of a successful ankle fusion. In addition, radiographic evidence of bridging trabeculae without failure of internal fixation or loss of correction is also a good sign of a successful ankle arthrodesis. Finally, CT scanning can be done if there is any doubt about a solid arthrodesis.[18] There are several reports on arthroscopic ankle fusion that show a mean time to union in 12 weeks after surgery.[3,19,20] The rate of union has been reported to range between 85% and 97%.[3,14,15,19–21]

The functional outcome of a particular technique is also extremely important. Many factors can come into play regarding the outcome, including fusion position, the mobility of adjacent joints, and metabolic bone issues, to name a few. Several studies have reported excellent results with arthroscopic ankle arthrodesis.[2,10,15,20,22] A meta-analysis of the literature regarding long-term outcomes of open ankle arthrodesis was performed in 2007. Haddad and colleagues[5] identified 39 primary studies that evaluated ankle arthrodesis in a total of 1262 patients. The results showed 31% excellent, 37% good, 13% fair, and 24% poor. The mean American Orthopaedic Foot and Ankle Society score was 75.6 points. Clearly, arthroscopic ankle arthrodesis seems to have equal or better outcomes when compared with open techniques.

SUMMARY

Arthroscopic ankle arthrodesis is a cost-effective option for many patients with post-traumatic arthritis of the ankle joint. Rehabilitation is generally quicker than conventional open techniques, and rates of fusion are comparable or better than traditional open techniques. Unless the arthroscopic surgeon has considerable experience, the best results are seen in patients with very little deformity in the ankle joint.

REFERENCES

1. O'Brien TS, Hart TS, Shereff MJ, et al. Open versus arthroscopic ankle arthrodesis: a comparative study. Foot Ankle Int 1990;20:368–74.
2. Myerson MS, Quil G. Ankle arthrodesis: a comparison of an arthroscopic and an open method of treatment. Clin Orthop 1991;268:85–95.
3. Winson IG, Robinson DE, Allen PE. Arthroscopic ankle arthrodesis. J Bone Joint Surg Br 2004;87(3):343–7.
4. DeHeer PA, Catorie SM, Taulman BB. Ankle arthrodesis: a literature review. Clin Podiatr Med Surg 2012;29(4):509–27.
5. Haddad SL, Coetzee JC, Estok R, et al. Intermediate and long-term outcomes of total ankle arthroplasty and ankle arthrodesis. A systematic review of the literature. J Bone Joint Surg Am 2007;89:1899–905.
6. Guyer AJ, Richardson EG. Current concepts review: total ankle arthroplasty. Foot Ankle Int 2008;29(2):256–64.
7. Bonnin M, Judet T, Colombier JA, et al. Midterm results of the Salto total ankle prosthesis. Clin Orthop 2004;424:6–18.
8. Henricson A, Skoog A, Carlsson A. The Swedish Ankle Arthroplasty Register: an analysis of 531 arthroplasties between 1993 and 2005. Acta Orthop 2007;78: 569–74.
9. Schneider D. Arthroscopic ankle fusion. Arthroscopic Video J 1983;3:35–47.
10. Zvijac JE, Lemak L, Schurhoff MR, et al. Analysis of arthroscopically assisted ankle arthrodesis. Arthroscopy 2002;18(1):70–5.
11. Peterson KS, Lee MS, Buddecke DE. Arthroscopic versus open ankle arthrodesis: a retrospective cost analysis. J Foot Ankle Surg 2010;49(3):242–7.
12. Nielsen KK, Linde F, Jensen NC. The outcome of arthroscopic and open surgery ankle arthrodesis: a comparative retrospective study of 107 patients. Foot Ankle Surg 2008;14(3):153–7.
13. Saltzman CL, Salamon ML, Blanchard GM, et al. Epidemiology of ankle arthritis. Report of a consecutive series of 639 patients from a tertiary orthopedic center. Iowa Orthop J 2005;25:44–6.
14. Gougoulias NE, Agathgelidis FG, Parsons SW. Arthroscopic ankle arthrodesis. Foot Ankle Int 2007;28(6):695–706.
15. Dannawi Z, Nawabi DH, Patel A, et al. Arthroscopic ankle arthrodesis: are results reproducible irrespective of preoperative deformity? Foot Ankle Surg 2011;17(4): 295–9.
16. Mazur JM, Schwartz E, Simon SR. Ankle arthrodesis: long-term follow-up with gait analysis. J Bone Joint Surg Am 1979;61:964–75.

17. Lynch AF, Bourne RB, Rorabeck CH. The long-term results of ankle arthrodesis. J Bone Joint Surg Br 1988;70:113–6.
18. Coughlin MJ, Grimes JS, Traughber PD, et al. Comparison of radiographs and CT scans in the prospective evaluation of the fusion of hindfoot arthrodesis. Foot Ankle Int 2006;27(10):780–7.
19. Pierre A, Hulet C, Locker B, et al. Arthroscopic tibia-talar arthrodesis: limitations and indications in 20 patients. Rev Chir Orthop Reparatrice Appar Mot 2003; 89(2):144–51.
20. Ferkel RD, Hewitt M. Long term results of arthroscopic ankle arthrodesis. Foot Ankle Int 2005;26(4):275–80.
21. Collman DR, Kass MH, Schuberth JM. Arthroscopic ankle arthrodesis: factors influencing union in 39 consecutive patients. Foot Ankle Int 2006;27(12):1079–85.
22. Kats J, Kampen A, Waal-Malefijt MC. Improvement in technique for arthroscopic ankle fusion: results in 15 patients. Knee Surg Sports Traumatol Arthrosc 2003; 11(1):46–9.

Index

Note: Page numbers of article titles are in **boldface** type.

Clin Podiatr Med Surg 33 (2016) 591–596
http://dx.doi.org/10.1016/S0891-8422(16)30087-8
0891-8422/16/$ – see front matter

podiatric.theclinics.com

UNITED STATES POSTAL SERVICE®

Statement of Ownership, Management, and Circulation
(All Periodicals Publications Except Requester Publications)

1. Publication Title	2. Publication Number	3. Filing Date
CLINICS IN PODIATRIC MEDICINE & SURGERY	000 – 707	9/18/2016

4. Issue Frequency	5. Number of Issues Published Annually	6. Annual Subscription Price
JAN, APR, JUL, OCT	4	$292.00

7. Complete Mailing Address of Known Office of Publication (Not printer) (Street, city, county, state, and ZIP+4®)

ELSEVIER INC.
360 PARK AVENUE SOUTH
NEW YORK, NY 10010-1710

Contact Person: STEPHEN R. BUSHING
Telephone (Include area code): 215-239-3688

8. Complete Mailing Address of Headquarters or General Business Office of Publisher (Not printer)

ELSEVIER INC.
360 PARK AVENUE SOUTH
NEW YORK, NY 10010-1710

9. Full Names and Complete Mailing Addresses of Publisher, Editor, and Managing Editor (Do not leave blank)

Publisher (Name and complete mailing address)

LINDA BELFUS, ELSEVIER INC.
1600 JOHN F KENNEDY BLVD. SUITE 1800
PHILADELPHIA, PA 19103-2899

Editor (Name and complete mailing address)

JENNIFER FLYNN-BRIGGS, ELSEVIER INC.
1600 JOHN F KENNEDY BLVD. SUITE 1800
PHILADELPHIA, PA 19103-2899

Managing Editor (Name and complete mailing address)

PATRICK J. MANLEY, JR.
1600 JOHN F KENNEDY BLVD. SUITE 1800
PHILADELPHIA, PA 19103-2899

10. Owner (Do not leave blank. If the publication is owned by a corporation, give the name and address of the corporation immediately followed by the names and addresses of all stockholders owning or holding 1 percent or more of the total amount of stock. If not owned by a corporation, give the names and addresses of the individual owners. If owned by a partnership or other unincorporated firm, give its name and address as well as those of each individual owner. If the publication is published by a nonprofit organization, give its name and address.)

Full Name	Complete Mailing Address
WHOLLY OWNED SUBSIDIARY OF REED/ELSEVIER US HOLDINGS	1600 JOHN F KENNEDY BLVD. SUITE 1800 PHILADELPHIA, PA 19103-2899

11. Known Bondholders, Mortgagees, and Other Security Holders Owning or Holding 1 Percent or More of Total Amount of Bonds, Mortgages, or Other Securities. If none, check box ▶ ☐ None

Full Name	Complete Mailing Address
N/A	

12. Tax Status (For completion by nonprofit organizations authorized to mail at nonprofit rates) (Check one)
The purpose, function, and nonprofit status of this organization and the exempt status for federal income tax purposes:
☐ Has Not Changed During Preceding 12 Months
☐ Has Changed During Preceding 12 Months (Publisher must submit explanation of change with this statement)

13. Publication Title	14. Issue Date for Circulation Data Below
CLINICS IN PODIATRIC MEDICINE & SURGERY	JULY 2016

PS Form 3526, July 2014 [Page 1 of 4 (see instructions page 4)] PSN: 7530-01-000-9931   PRIVACY NOTICE: See our privacy policy on www.usps.com.

15. Extent and Nature of Circulation			Average No. Copies Each Issue During Preceding 12 Months	No. Copies of Single Issue Published Nearest to Filing Date
a. Total Number of Copies (Net press run)			283	317
b. Paid Circulation (By Mail and Outside the Mail)	(1)	Mailed Outside-County Paid Subscriptions Stated on PS Form 3541 (Include paid distribution above nominal rate, advertiser's proof copies, and exchange copies)	159	192
	(2)	Mailed In-County Paid Subscriptions Stated on PS Form 3541 (Include paid distribution above nominal rate, advertiser's proof copies, and exchange copies)	0	0
	(3)	Paid Distribution Outside the Mails Including Sales Through Dealers and Carriers, Street Vendors, Counter Sales, and Other Paid Distribution Outside USPS®	17	21
	(4)	Paid Distribution by Other Classes of Mail Through the USPS (e.g., First-Class Mail®)	0	0
c. Total Paid Distribution (Sum of 15b (1), (2), (3), and (4))			176	213
d. Free or Nominal Rate Distribution (By Mail and Outside the Mail)	(1)	Free or Nominal Rate Outside-County Copies included on PS Form 3541	53	64
	(2)	Free or Nominal Rate In-County Copies Included on PS Form 3541	0	0
	(3)	Free or Nominal Rate Copies Mailed at Other Classes Through the USPS (e.g., First-Class Mail)	0	0
	(4)	Free or Nominal Rate Distribution Outside the Mail (Carriers or other means)	0	0
e. Total Free or Nominal Rate Distribution (Sum of 15d (1), (2), (3) and (4))			53	64
f. Total Distribution (Sum of 15c and 15e)			229	277
g. Copies not Distributed (See Instructions to Publishers #4 (page 3))			54	40
h. Total (Sum of 15f and g)			283	317
i. Percent Paid (15c divided by 15f times 100)			77%	77%

* If you are claiming electronic copies, go to line 16 on page 3. If you are not claiming electronic copies, skip to line 17 on page 3.

16. Electronic Copy Circulation	Average No. Copies Each Issue During Preceding 12 Months	No. Copies of Single Issue Published Nearest to Filing Date
a. Paid Electronic Copies ▶	0	0
b. Total Paid Print Copies (Line 15c) + Paid Electronic Copies (Line 16a) ▶	176	213
c. Total Print Distribution (Line 15f) + Paid Electronic Copies (Line 16a) ▶	229	277
d. Percent Paid (Both Print & Electronic Copies) (16b divided by 16c × 100) ▶	77%	77%

☒ I certify that 50% of all my distributed copies (electronic and print) are paid above a nominal price.

17. Publication of Statement of Ownership

☒ If the publication is a general publication, publication of this statement is required. Will be printed ☐ Publication not required.

in the OCTOBER 2016 issue of this publication.

18. Signature and Title of Editor, Publisher, Business Manager, or Owner

STEPHEN R. BUSHING - INVENTORY DISTRIBUTION CONTROL MANAGER

Date 9/18/2016

I certify that all information furnished on this form is true and complete. I understand that anyone who furnishes false or misleading information on this form or who omits material or information requested on the form may be subject to criminal sanctions (including fines and imprisonment) and/or civil sanctions (including civil penalties).

PS Form 3526, July 2014 (Page 3 of 4)   PRIVACY NOTICE: See our privacy policy on www.usps.com.

Moving?

Make sure your subscription moves with you!

To notify us of your new address, find your **Clinics Account Number** (located on your mailing label above your name), and contact customer service at:

Email: journalscustomerservice-usa@elsevier.com

800-654-2452 (subscribers in the U.S. & Canada)
314-447-8871 (subscribers outside of the U.S. & Canada)

Fax number: 314-447-8029

Elsevier Health Sciences Division
Subscription Customer Service
3251 Riverport Lane
Maryland Heights, MO 63043

*To ensure uninterrupted delivery of your subscription, please notify us at least 4 weeks in advance of move.

Printed and bound by CPI Group (UK) Ltd, Croydon, CR0 4YY

03/10/2024

01040388-0009